The complete chair yoga for seniors

The ultimate guide to enhance flexibility, strength and inner peace with mindfulness practices for a healthier and happy lifestyle

George Brian

Table of content

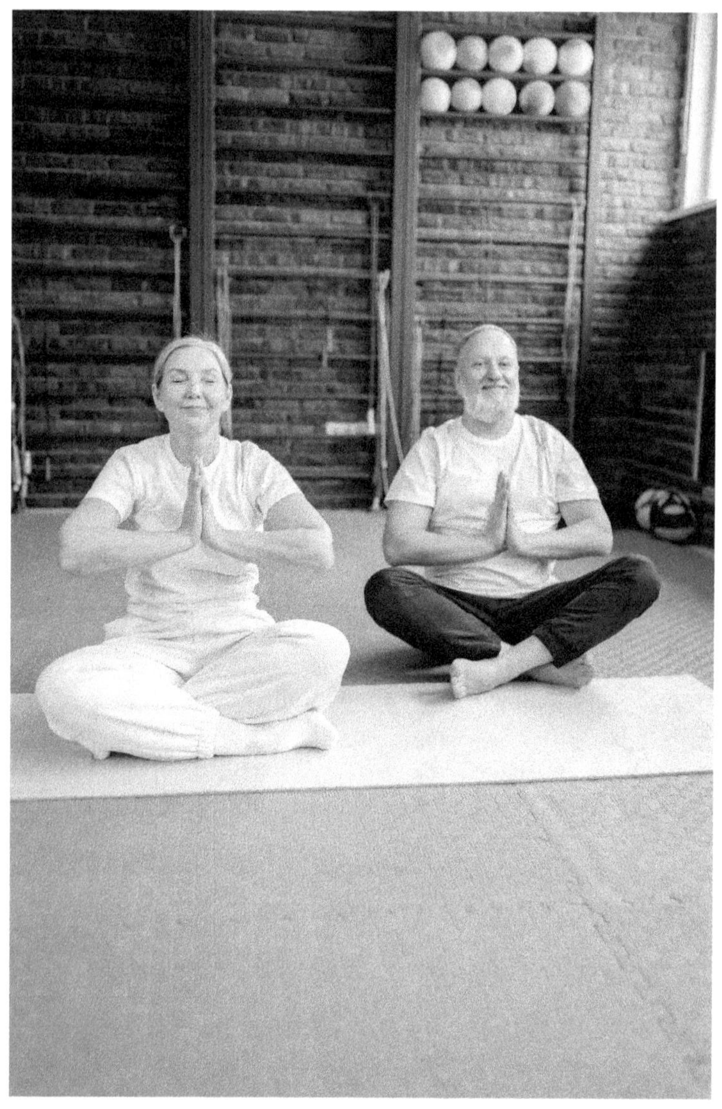

INTRODUCTION

UNDERSTANDING CHAIR YOGA

Chair yoga is a modified form of traditional yoga that adapts traditional yoga poses for people to practice while sitting in a chair. It is designed to be gentle, accessible, and beneficial for individuals with limited mobility, chronic pain, or other health conditions. Some of the key aspects of chair yoga include:

- **Benefits:** Regular practice of chair yoga can help increase flexibility, improve mobility, and benefit cardiovascular health. It is also known to promote flexibility, strength, and manage stress and anxiety

- **Accessibility:** Chair yoga is suitable for people of all ages and fitness levels, making it an excellent option for seniors, individuals with physical limitations, or those who prefer a low-impact form of exercise

- **Equipment:** A yoga chair, which has a higher backrest and a wider seat than a regular chair, is used for chair yoga

- **Sequence:** Chair yoga sequences can be as short as 10 minutes or as long as an hour, depending on your needs and preferences. They often include breathing exercises, gentle stretches, and simple yoga poses

- **Instructors:** If you are new to chair yoga, it is recommended to take a few classes with a certified instructor to learn the proper techniques and poses. You can find chair yoga classes at local yoga studios or online

Chair Yoga Poses

Some simple and effective chair yoga exercises include

1. **Sitting in the chair:** Sit upright with your feet flat on the floor and your hands resting on your thighs or knees.

2. **Breathing exercises:** Practice deep breathing, taking slow and steady breaths in and out through your nose.

3. **Gentle stretches:** Reach your arms overhead, stretch your legs out in front of

you, or gently twist your torso from side to side.

4. **Simple poses:** Perform poses such as the chair pose, warrior II, or tree pose, adapted to be done while sitting in the chair.

Remember to listen to your body and stop any pose if it causes pain or discomfort. Chair yoga is meant to be a gentle exercise that helps you gain flexibility, strength, and manage stress and anxiety

Principles of Chair Yoga

Chair yoga adapts traditional yoga poses to be performed while seated. The principles of chair yoga revolve around accessibility, adaptability, and mindfulness.

1 Accessibility: Chair yoga makes the benefits of yoga accessible to a broader audience, including those with mobility issues, seniors, or individuals with physical limitations. The use of a chair provides stability and support, making it possible for people who may struggle with floor-based yoga to participate.

2 **Adaptability:** Chair yoga is highly adaptable, allowing individuals to modify poses based on their abilities and comfort level. This flexibility makes it suitable for various fitness levels and health conditions. Poses can be adjusted to accommodate different ranges of motion, ensuring inclusivity.

3 **Mindfulness:** Like traditional yoga, chair yoga emphasizes mindfulness and conscious breathing. Participants are encouraged to focus on the present moment, promoting relaxation, stress reduction, and mental well-being. The integration of breathwork enhances the mind-body connection.

4 **Gentle Movement:** The principles of chair yoga prioritize gentle movements that promote flexibility and joint health. This approach reduces the risk of strain or injury, making it suitable for individuals recovering from injuries or dealing with chronic conditions such as arthritis.

5 **Seated Postures:** Since participants are seated throughout the practice, chair yoga focuses on developing strength and flexibility while seated. This is particularly beneficial for those who may have difficulty getting up and down from the floor, allowing them to experience the benefits of yoga without the need for transitions between standing and seated postures.

6 Breath-Centered Practice: Chair yoga places a significant emphasis on breath awareness. Through specific breathing exercises, individuals learn to control and deepen their breath, promoting relaxation and improving respiratory function. The breath becomes a focal point for mindfulness and stress management.

7 Promoting Circulation: The gentle movements in chair yoga can help improve circulation, especially in the legs and feet. This is particularly important for individuals with sedentary lifestyles or those with limited mobility.

8 Community and Social Connection: Chair yoga classes often foster a sense of community and social connection. Participants can engage in a supportive and inclusive environment, sharing their experiences and building connections with others.

9 Therapeutic Benefits: Chair yoga is increasingly recognized for its therapeutic benefits. It can be used as a complementary approach to manage various health conditions, including chronic pain, hypertension, and stress-related disorders. The gentle nature of the practice makes it suitable for rehabilitation purposes as well.

The principles of chair yoga center around making the practice accessible to a diverse population, emphasizing adaptability, promoting mindfulness through breath awareness, incorporating gentle movements, and fostering a sense of community and well-being.

Adaptability for Seniors

Adaptability in chair yoga for seniors is crucial to ensure a safe and enjoyable practice. Seniors often face various physical limitations, such as reduced flexibility, joint issues, or balance concerns. To address these challenges, chair yoga emphasizes adaptability in poses and movements.

1 Seated Poses:

- Incorporate a variety of seated poses that cater to different levels of flexibility.
- Modify traditional yoga poses to be performed comfortably while seated on a chair.
- Encourage seniors to focus on proper alignment and breath control, promoting relaxation and stress reduction.

2 Gentle Stretches:

- Integrate gentle stretches to improve flexibility without straining joints.
- Emphasize controlled movements, allowing seniors to gradually increase their range of motion.
- Provide modifications for each stretch, accommodating individuals with varying degrees of flexibility.

3 Chair Support:

- Utilize the chair as a stable prop for balance and support during standing poses.
- Teach seniors to use the chair for stability when transitioning between poses, minimizing the risk of falls.
- Ensure that the chair is positioned securely, promoting a sense of confidence and safety.

4 Breathing Exercises:

- Include breath awareness exercises to enhance lung capacity and reduce stress.
- Emphasize the importance of slow, deep breaths to calm the nervous system.
- Adapt breathing techniques to accommodate any respiratory challenges seniors may face.

5   Mindful Movement:

- Encourage a mindful approach to movement, fostering a connection between the body and mind.
- Emphasize the importance of listening to one's body and modifying poses accordingly.
- Incorporate guided meditation or visualization to enhance the overall experience.

6   Customization for Health Conditions:

- Tailor chair yoga routines to address specific health concerns such as arthritis, osteoporosis, or cardiovascular issues.
- Provide alternatives for individuals with limited mobility or chronic pain.
- Educate seniors about the benefits of chair yoga in managing and improving various health conditions.

7   Community Engagement:

- Foster a supportive community environment where seniors feel comfortable sharing their concerns and progress.
- Modify exercises based on individual feedback and needs, creating a personalized and inclusive practice.

- Offer variations to accommodate different fitness levels within the senior group.

8 Regular Progress Assessments:

- Conduct regular assessments to track progress and adapt the chair yoga routine accordingly.
- Adjust difficulty levels based on the evolving capabilities of the participants.
- Celebrate achievements, reinforcing a positive and motivating atmosphere.

By prioritizing adaptability in chair yoga for seniors, instructors can create a holistic and inclusive practice that promotes physical well-being, mental relaxation, and a sense of community among participants.

BENEFITS AND CONSIDERATIONS

Benefits of Chair Yoga for Seniors:

Improved Flexibility:

Chair yoga incorporates gentle stretches, enhancing flexibility in seniors, making daily movements easier and reducing stiffness.

Strength Building:

The use of resistance in chair yoga exercises helps seniors build muscle strength, supporting overall mobility and stability.

Enhanced Circulation:

Controlled movements and deep breathing stimulate blood flow, improving circulation and potentially benefiting cardiovascular health in seniors.

Stress Reduction:

Chair yoga emphasizes relaxation techniques, including deep breathing and meditation, aiding seniors in managing stress and promoting mental well-being.

Joint Health:

The low-impact nature of chair yoga is gentle on joints, making it suitable for individuals with arthritis or other joint conditions, promoting joint health.

Improved Posture:

Chair yoga includes exercises that promote better posture, addressing common issues related to aging and prolonged periods of sitting.

Mind-Body Connection:

Incorporating mindfulness practices, chair yoga fosters a strong mind-body connection, enhancing mental clarity, focus, and overall cognitive well-being.

Social Engagement:

Participating in chair yoga classes provides seniors with a social outlet, fostering a sense of community, reducing feelings of isolation, and promoting mental health.

Considerations for Complete Chair Yoga for Seniors:

Health Assessment:

Seniors should undergo a thorough health assessment before starting chair yoga, identifying any pre-existing conditions or physical limitations.

Qualified Instructors:

Ensure chair yoga classes are led by instructors with expertise in working with seniors, understanding their unique needs and providing appropriate guidance.

Adaptability:

Chair yoga routines should be adaptable, considering varying fitness levels and accommodating participants with different mobility levels.

Individualized Approach:

Tailor chair yoga sessions to address individual health concerns, providing modifications as needed to accommodate participants' specific requirements.

Communication:

Establish open lines of communication between seniors and instructors, encouraging participants to express any discomfort or concerns during the practice.

Safety First:

Emphasize safety precautions, such as using sturdy chairs and avoiding positions that may strain joints, ensuring a safe environment for seniors to practice.

Gradual Progression:

Seniors should progress gradually in chair yoga, avoiding overexertion and allowing time for adaptation to new movements and postures.

Medical Clearance:

Seniors with chronic health conditions should seek medical clearance before beginning chair yoga, ensuring compatibility with their overall health and any necessary adjustments to the practice.

Chair yoga for seniors offers a comprehensive range of physical and mental benefits, but a thoughtful and individualized approach, coupled with qualified instruction and attention to safety, is crucial for a successful and enjoyable practice.

Positive Impacts on Physical Health

Chair yoga for seniors encompasses a range of positive impacts on physical health, providing a tailored and accessible approach to exercise for older individuals. Let's delve into the details:

1 Flexibility and Range of Motion:

- Chair yoga incorporates gentle stretches and movements that target various muscle groups, promoting flexibility.

- Seniors can maintain or improve their range of motion, reducing stiffness and enhancing joint flexibility.
- This is particularly beneficial for daily activities, such as reaching, bending, and turning, contributing to overall mobility.

2 Strength Building:

- Focusing on muscles crucial for stability and balance, chair yoga helps seniors build and maintain strength.
- The use of a chair as a prop ensures stability, making it accessible for those with mobility challenges or limited strength.
- Improved strength contributes to better stability, reducing the risk of falls and injuries.

3 Posture Enhancement:

- Emphasizing proper alignment during poses, chair yoga supports seniors in improving and maintaining good posture.
- Enhanced posture not only reduces strain on the spine but also facilitates proper breathing patterns.
- This is essential for spinal health and can alleviate discomfort associated with poor posture.

4 Breathing Techniques and Lung Capacity:

- Chair yoga incorporates mindful breathing techniques that focus on deep, controlled breaths.
- This improves lung capacity, enhancing oxygenation throughout the body.
- Proper breathing has positive effects on cardiovascular health, supporting heart function and overall well-being.

5 Stress Reduction and Relaxation:

- The relaxation elements of chair yoga create a meditative and calming environment.
- Seniors can release tension, leading to reduced stress levels.
- Chronic stress reduction can positively impact blood pressure, immune function, and mental well-being.

6 Circulation Improvement:

- Gentle movements and stretches in chair yoga contribute to improved circulation.
- This can help alleviate issues like swelling in the extremities, promoting better blood flow.
- Enhanced circulation supports cardiovascular health, reducing the risk of conditions like hypertension.

7 Low-Impact and Inclusivity:

- Chair yoga is a low-impact exercise, making it suitable for seniors with various health conditions or physical limitations.
- The accessibility of chair yoga encourages regular participation, fostering a consistent exercise routine.
- This inclusivity promotes overall health and well-being for a diverse senior population.

Chair yoga for seniors offers a comprehensive and nuanced approach to physical health. From promoting flexibility and strength to enhancing posture, breathing, and circulation, chair yoga provides a holistic and accessible avenue for older individuals to maintain and improve their overall well-being. Regular engagement in chair yoga can empower seniors to lead active, balanced, and healthy lives.

Enhancing Mental Well-being

Chair yoga is a gentle form of yoga that can be adapted to accommodate seniors, promoting physical and mental well-being. Here's a detailed guide to enhancing mental well-being through a complete chair yoga routine for seniors:

1   Start with Mindful Breathing:

Begin the session with deep, mindful breathing exercises. Inhale slowly, expanding the diaphragm, and exhale fully. Emphasize the importance of being present in the moment.

2   Neck and Shoulder Stretches:

- Gently move the head from side to side and in circular motions to release tension in the neck.
- Encourage seniors to roll their shoulders backward and forward, promoting relaxation and improved blood circulation.

3   Seated Cat-Cow Stretch:

- Guide participants through a seated version of the cat-cow stretch, arching and rounding the spine to enhance flexibility and stimulate the spine.

4   Chair Pigeon Pose:

- Engage in a modified pigeon pose by crossing one ankle over the opposite knee

while seated. This helps stretch the hips
and lower back, easing any discomfort.

5 Seated Forward Bend:

- Instruct seniors to hinge at the hips and
  reach forward, keeping the back straight.
  This gentle forward bend can alleviate
  tension in the spine and promote relaxation.

6 Twisting Chair Pose:

- Guide participants in a seated twist,
  encouraging them to hold onto the back of
  the chair for support. Twists help improve
  digestion and release tension in the spine.

7 Mindful Meditation:

- Introduce a brief meditation session,
  focusing on mindfulness and present
  awareness. Use calming cues to guide
  seniors through a relaxed state of mind.

8 Chair Yoga Nidra:

- Incorporate a short Yoga Nidra session, a
  form of guided relaxation. This can help
  seniors experience a deep state of
  relaxation and reduce stress.

9 Balance Exercises:

- Include seated balance exercises to improve stability and concentration. For example, lifting one foot at a time or extending the legs while maintaining posture.

10 Closing Savasana:

- Conclude the chair yoga session with a seated Savasana, allowing seniors to relax and absorb the benefits of the practice. Encourage them to focus on their breath and let go of any remaining tension.

11 Positive Affirmations:

- End the session with positive affirmations, fostering a positive mindset and emotional well-being. Encourage participants to express gratitude and kindness towards themselves.

Remember to tailor the routine to the participants' abilities and ensure they feel comfortable throughout the session. Regular practice of this chair yoga routine can contribute significantly to the mental well-being of seniors by promoting relaxation, mindfulness, and a sense of connection between the body and mind.

Chapter One

GETTING STARTED WITH CHAIR YOGA

Choosing the Right Chair

Selecting the right chair for complete chair yoga for seniors involves considerations specific to their comfort, safety, and ease of movement. Here are key factors to keep in mind:

1 Stability and Support:

- Opt for a chair with a sturdy frame to provide stability during yoga poses.
- Look for a chair with a high backrest for added support, especially when seniors are transitioning between poses.

2 Comfortable Seat:

- Choose a chair with a comfortable, well-padded seat to enhance comfort during seated poses.
- Ensure the seat is wide enough for seniors to sit comfortably without feeling restricted.

3 Adjustability:

- Consider chairs with adjustable features like seat height and armrests to accommodate different body types and preferences.
- Adjustable armrests are beneficial for modifying poses and adapting to individual needs.

4 Non-Slip Base:

- Ensure the chair has a non-slip base to prevent sliding or tipping during yoga movements.
- Rubberized or gripped feet add an extra layer of safety, especially on smooth surfaces.

5 Armrests:

- While some poses benefit from armrests, others may require more freedom of movement. Choose a chair with removable or adjustable armrests to cater to various yoga positions.

6 Space Efficiency:

- Consider the available space for performing chair yoga. A chair that allows ample room for movement without obstruction is essential.
- Foldable or stackable chairs can be convenient for storage when not in use.

7 Material:

- Opt for a chair with a breathable material to prevent discomfort during longer yoga sessions.
- Chairs with easy-to-clean materials are practical for maintaining hygiene.

8 Ease of Access:

- Seniors should be able to get in and out of the chair with ease. Choose a chair with an appropriate height and armrest design to facilitate smooth transitions.

9 Wheelchair Accessibility:

- For seniors using wheelchairs, ensure the chosen chair complements their mobility device. It should provide a stable surface for

yoga practice without compromising
wheelchair accessibility.

10 Instructional Support:

- Some chairs designed for senior yoga come
  with instructional materials or DVDs. These
  can guide seniors through poses and
  ensure they practice safely and effectively.

11 Reviews and Recommendations:

- Research reviews from other seniors or
  yoga instructors specializing in chair yoga.
- Recommendations from healthcare
  professionals or yoga instructors
  experienced in working with seniors can
  offer valuable insights.

By carefully considering these factors, you can
choose a chair that enhances the chair yoga
experience for seniors, promoting physical
well-being, flexibility, and overall health.

Criteria for an Ideal Chair

An ideal chair encompasses a multifaceted set of criteria, ranging from ergonomic considerations to design aesthetics. Let's delve into these criteria more extensively:

1 Ergonomics:

- **Back Support:** An ideal chair should offer adequate lumbar support, maintaining the natural curve of the spine. Adjustable lumbar support allows users to customize it based on their unique needs.
- **Seat Design:** The seat should be contoured to distribute weight evenly, preventing discomfort or pressure points. Adjustable seat height is essential for accommodating various body types and ensuring proper alignment with work surfaces.
- **Armrests:** Adjustable and padded armrests contribute to optimal arm and shoulder support. They should align comfortably with the user's desk or work surface.

2 Materials and Durability:

- **Quality Materials:** The chair should be crafted from durable and high-quality materials, ensuring longevity and resilience to wear and tear.

- **Upholstery:** The choice of upholstery matters for both comfort and aesthetics. Breathable, easy-to-clean fabrics enhance user experience and maintenance.

3 Comfort:

- **Padding:** Ample padding, especially in the seat and backrest, enhances overall comfort during prolonged use.
- **Reclining and Tilt Mechanism:** A chair that allows for reclining or tilting provides users with flexibility and the ability to change positions for increased comfort.

4 Adjustability:

- **Customization Options:** Adjustable features, including seat height, armrest height, and tilt tension, enable users to tailor the chair to their specific needs and preferences.
- **Swivel and Casters:** 360-degree swivel and smooth-rolling casters promote mobility and ease of movement, contributing to user convenience.

5 Sturdiness and Stability:

- **Frame Construction:** A robust frame ensures the chair's stability and longevity.

The chair should withstand daily use without compromising its structural integrity.

6 Functionality:

- **Versatility:** An ideal chair should be versatile, suitable for various settings such as offices, homes, or public spaces.
- **Storage Features:** Additional features like built-in storage or side pockets enhance functionality, providing convenient storage for small items.

7 Aesthetic Considerations:

- **Design Cohesiveness:** The chair's design should complement the overall aesthetic of its surroundings, whether in a modern office space or a classic home environment.
- **Color and Style:** Aesthetic appeal is subjective, but a well-designed chair should have a visually pleasing color scheme and style.

An ideal chair integrates ergonomic principles, durable materials, comfort-enhancing features, adjustability, stability, versatility, and aesthetic considerations to create a comprehensive and user-centric seating solution. This holistic approach ensures that the chair not only meets practical needs but also enhances the overall user experience.

Types of Chairs for Different Needs

1. **Ergonomic Office Chairs:**

   - Designed for extended periods of sitting.
   - Provides lumbar support for lower back comfort.
   - Adjustable features cater to individual preferences.

2. **Accent Chairs:**

   - Adds style to a room while offering comfortable seating.
   - Comes in various designs and materials to suit decor.

3. **Wingback Chairs:**

   - Features "wings" on the sides for head and neck support.
   - Classic design with a touch of elegance.

4. **Club Chairs:**

- Upholstered, typically with a lower back and arms.
- Well-padded for comfort, often found in living rooms.

5. **Adirondack Chairs:**

- Outdoor chairs with a slanted back and wide armrests.
- Perfect for relaxation on a patio or in a garden.

6. **Rocking Chairs:**

- Provides a soothing rocking motion.
- Popular for nurseries or relaxation spaces.

7. **Chaise Lounge Chairs:**

- Long chair for reclining or lounging.
- Often found in bedrooms or as part of outdoor furniture.

8. **Folding Chairs:**

- Convenient for temporary seating needs.
- Compact and easy to store or transport.

9. Armchairs:

- Upholstered chairs with armrests.
- Adaptable and suitable for a range of environments.

10. Gaming Chairs:

- Designed for prolonged gaming sessions.
- Often features ergonomic design and built-in technology.

11. Dining Chairs:

- Accompanies dining tables.
- Available in various styles, materials, and heights.

12. Swivel Chairs:

- Rotates on a base for easy movement.
- Suitable for office use or as accent furniture.

13. Lounge Chairs:

- Low-slung, relaxed seating.
- Perfect for casual and comfortable environments.

14. Armless Chairs:

- Streamlined design without armrests.
- Fits well in smaller spaces and modern settings.

15. High-Backed Chairs:

- Offers support for the upper back.
- Adds a sense of privacy and comfort.

16. Zero Gravity Chairs:

- Reclines to a position that minimizes stress on the spine.
- Promotes a feeling of weightlessness and relaxation.

17. Bucket Chairs:

- Shaped like a bucket for a snug seating experience.
- Modern design with a cozy feel.

18. Ball Chairs:

- Features an exercise ball as the seat.

- Encourages core engagement and better posture.

19. Acoustic Chairs:

- Designed for optimal sound absorption.
- Ideal for creating quiet, focused spaces.

20. Convertible Chairs:

- Adaptable for different functions (e.g., sofa to bed).
- Maximizes versatility in limited spaces.

Choosing the right chair involves considering functionality, comfort, and aesthetics based on individual needs and the intended use of the chair.

WARM-UP AND PRECAUTIONS

Warm-up and precautions are crucial aspects of any exercise routine, including chair yoga for seniors. Here's a comprehensive guide:

Warm-up for Chair Yoga:

1. **Neck Stretches:**
   - Gently turn your head from side to side.
   - Drop your ear towards each shoulder.
   - Slowly roll your neck in both directions.

2. **Shoulder Rolls:**
   - Lift your shoulders up towards your ears, then roll them backward and downward.
   - Repeat in the forward direction.

3. **Arm Stretches:**
   - Extend your arms straight out, then bring them overhead and back down.
   - Rotate your wrists and make circular motions with your arms.

4. **Spinal Flexibility:**
   - Sit tall and twist gently from side to side.
   - Breathe in as you extend your back and out as you bend.

5. **Seated Cat-Cow Stretch:**
   - Arch your back on the inhale, bringing your chest forward.
   - Round your back on the exhale, bringing your chin to your chest.

6. **Hip Openers:**
   - Raising your knees toward your chest one at a time.
   - Make circular motions with your knees.

7. **Ankle Rolls:**
   - Lift one foot at a time and rotate your ankle in both directions.

8. **Deep Breathing:**
   - Inhale deeply through your nose, expanding your belly.
   - Exhale slowly through pursed lips.

Precautions for Chair Yoga

1 **Consult with a Healthcare Professional:**

Before starting any exercise program, seniors should consult their healthcare provider to ensure chair yoga is suitable for their individual health condition.

2 Chair Stability:

Ensure that the chair is stable and placed
on a non-slip surface to prevent accidents
during movements.

3 Comfortable Clothing:

Dress comfortably with loose-fitting apparel
that doesn't restrict your movement.

4 Modify Poses as Needed:

Seniors should feel free to modify poses
based on their comfort level. If a pose
causes discomfort or pain, it should be
adjusted or skipped.

5 Mindful Movement:

Emphasize slow and controlled movements
to avoid sudden jerks or overexertion.

6 Breathing Awareness:

Focus on conscious breathing throughout
the session to enhance relaxation and
reduce stress.

7 Limit Range of Motion:

Be cautious not to overextend joints. Keep movements within a comfortable range to prevent injuries.

8 Hydration:

Stay well-hydrated before, during, and after the session.

9 Monitoring Heart Rate:

Seniors should monitor their heart rate and modify the intensity if needed, especially if they have cardiovascular concerns.

10 Rest Periods:

Encourage participants to take breaks and rest whenever needed. Overexertion should be avoided.

By incorporating these warm-up exercises and precautions, seniors can enjoy the benefits of chair yoga safely, promoting flexibility, balance, and overall well-being.

Importance of Proper Warm-up

1. **Enhanced Blood Circulation:**

    - Proper warm-up increases blood flow to muscles and joints.
    - Improved circulation ensures that the muscles receive an adequate supply of oxygen and nutrients.
    - This heightened blood flow is crucial for seniors, promoting flexibility and reducing the risk of muscle strains.

2. **Joint Lubrication and Flexibility:**

    - Aging can lead to a decrease in synovial fluid in joints.
    - Warm-up exercises, especially joint rotations and gentle stretches, help lubricate the joints.
    - Improved joint lubrication enhances flexibility, making it easier for seniors to move into various chair yoga poses.

3. **Muscle Preparation and Relaxation:**

    - Gradual warm-up prepares muscles for more intense activity.
    - Warm muscles are less likely to get injured and more flexible.

- This phase also allows for mental relaxation, reducing tension and anxiety associated with physical activity.

4. Injury Prevention:

- Seniors may have underlying health conditions or reduced bone density, making injury prevention crucial.
- A proper warm-up gradually increases heart rate and body temperature, preparing the body for the demands of chair yoga.
- It reduces the risk of strains, sprains, and other injuries, ensuring a safer practice.

5. Improved Range of Motion:

- Age-related stiffness can limit the range of motion in joints.
- Warm-up exercises target specific muscle groups, enhancing flexibility and increasing the range of motion.
- This is particularly important for seniors who may face challenges in movement due to conditions like arthritis.

6. **Balance and Coordination:**

- Aging can impair coordination and balance, which raises the possibility of falls.
- Warm-up routines that incorporate balance exercises help seniors improve stability.
- Improved balance is essential for chair yoga poses that may involve subtle weight shifts or changes in body alignment.

7. **Mind-Body Connection:**

- Warm-up fosters a connection between the mind and body.
- Mindful breathing exercises during warm-up contribute to mental preparedness.
- Seniors can approach chair yoga with increased awareness, promoting a more satisfying and meditative practice.

8. **Tailored Warm-Up for Seniors:**

- A well-designed warm-up takes into account the specific needs of seniors.

- Seated exercises, gentle stretches, and controlled movements are tailored to accommodate potential limitations.
- This customization ensures that the warm-up is accessible and beneficial for older individuals.

The importance of a proper warm-up for chair yoga in seniors lies in its multifaceted benefits. From physical preparation to mental readiness, a thorough warm-up sets the stage for a safe, enjoyable, and effective chair yoga practice for seniors, contributing to their overall health and well-being.

Safety Precautions and Consultations

When conducting chair yoga for seniors, prioritizing safety is crucial. Begin by ensuring that participants have medical clearance from their healthcare providers to engage in physical activity. Tailor the chair yoga routine to accommodate individual abilities and health conditions. Emphasize the following safety precautions and consultations:

1 **Health Screenings:**

- Before starting chair yoga, seniors should undergo health screenings to identify any underlying conditions or limitations.
- Encourage participants to communicate openly about their health history, injuries, or concerns.

2 **Professional Consultations:**

- Advocate for seniors to consult with their physicians or healthcare professionals before joining chair yoga sessions, especially if they have chronic illnesses or recent surgeries.

3 **Individualized Modifications:**

- Provide personalized modifications for poses to accommodate varying levels of flexibility, strength, and mobility among participants.
- Emphasize the importance of listening to their bodies and not pushing beyond their comfort zones.

4 **Clear Communication:**

- Maintain open communication channels with participants to address any discomfort or pain they may experience during the session.

- Encourage them to ask questions and express their needs for modifications.

5 Proper Warm-up and Cool Down:

- Incorporate gentle warm-up exercises to prepare muscles and joints for movement, reducing the risk of strains.
- Include a structured cool-down segment to help participants gradually return to a resting state and prevent abrupt changes in heart rate.

6 Stable Seating Arrangements:

- Ensure that participants have sturdy and stable chairs without wheels, ensuring a secure foundation for the exercises.
- Check the condition of chairs regularly to prevent accidents.

7 Balance and Stability Focus:

- Integrate exercises that enhance balance and stability to reduce the risk of falls, a common concern for seniors.
- Use the chair as a support when necessary, allowing participants to build confidence gradually.

8 Awareness of Physical Limitations:

- Instruct participants to be mindful of their physical limitations and to avoid overexertion.
- Encourage self-awareness and body awareness to prevent injury.

9 Hydration:

- Remind participants to stay hydrated throughout the session, as proper hydration is essential for overall well-being.

10 Emergency Preparedness:

- Be prepared for emergencies by having basic first aid knowledge and access to emergency contact information for each participant.
- Create a safe environment, free from obstacles and hazards.

By implementing these safety precautions and consultations, chair yoga sessions for seniors can be enjoyable, beneficial, and most importantly, conducted with their well-being in mind.

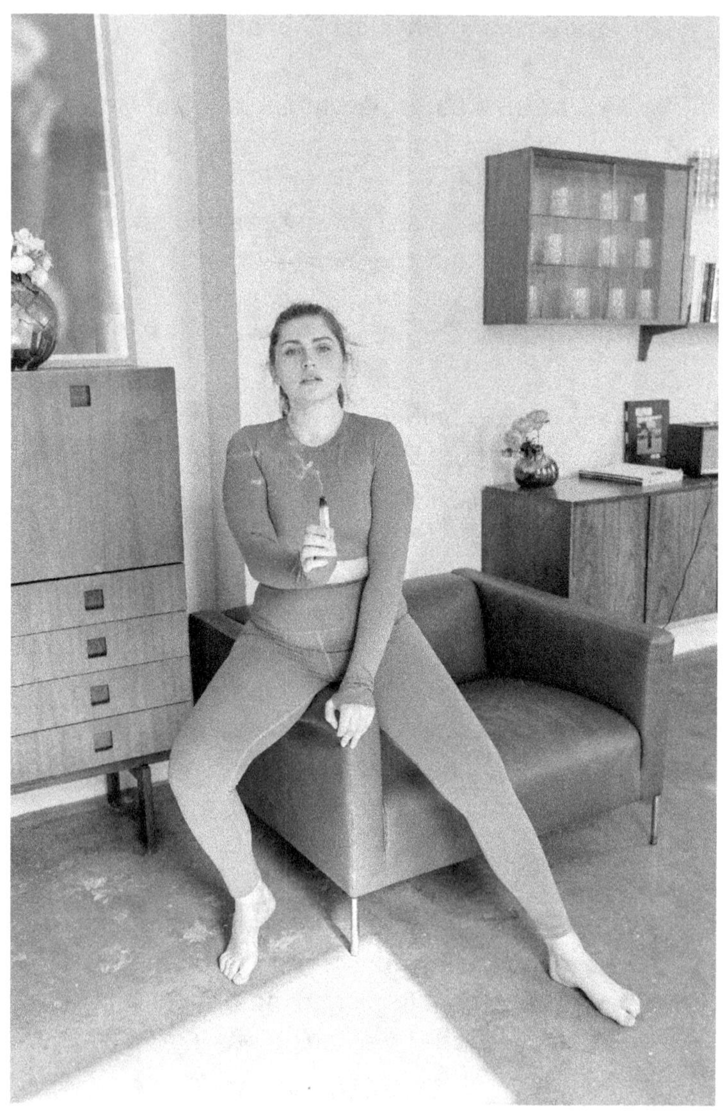

Chapter Two

SEATED POSES FOR SENIORS

Gentle Neck and Shoulder Practices

Here are detailed instructions for gentle neck and shoulder practices in a complete chair yoga routine for seniors:

1. **Neck Tilts:**

   - Maintain a straight spine while sitting comfortably in a chair.
   - Inhale and gently tilt your head to one side, bringing your ear towards your shoulder.
   - Exhale and return to the center.
   - Repeat on the other side.
   - Continue this gentle tilting motion, allowing your neck muscles to stretch with each movement.

2. Neck Rotations:

- Inhale and slowly rotate your head to the right, bringing your chin towards your chest and then to the left.
- Exhale and complete the circle, maintaining a smooth and controlled pace.
- Repeat in the opposite direction.
- Focus on the full range of motion, but only move as far as is comfortable.

3. Shoulder Rolls:

- As you inhale, raise your shoulders to your ears.
- Exhale and roll your shoulders back and down in a smooth, circular motion.
- Repeat this rolling motion several times.
- Then, reverse the direction, rolling your shoulders forward.
- This aids in releasing upper back and shoulder strain.

4. Seated Cat-Cow Stretches:

- Inhale and arch your back, lifting your chest and chin slightly.

- Breathe out, arch your back, and bring your chin up to your chest.
- Repeat this seated cat-cow flow, coordinating breath with movement.
- Feel the gentle stretch along your neck and upper back.

5. Seated Spinal Twists:

- Inhale, lengthen your spine, and exhale as you twist gently to one side.
- Hold the twist for a few breaths, feeling the stretch in your neck and upper back.
- Repeat on the other side, then inhale back to the center.
- Maintain a slow and controlled pace, avoiding any sudden movements.

6. Eagle Arms:

- Extend your arms forward at shoulder height.
- Cross your right arm under the left, intertwining your wrists.
- Raise your elbows just enough to feel a stretch in your shoulders and upper back.
- Hold for a few breaths, then release and switch arms.

7. Side Bends and Lateral Stretches:

- Inhale and lift your arms overhead.
- Exhale and gently lean to one side, feeling the stretch along your side and shoulder.
- Continue these lateral stretches, promoting flexibility in the neck and shoulders.

8. Neck and Shoulder Self-Massage:

- Use your fingertips to massage the base of your skull and neck in gentle circular motions.
- Apply light pressure to the shoulders and upper back, releasing tension.
- Encourage seniors to explore areas of discomfort and massage as needed, being mindful of their own comfort levels.

9. Relaxation:

- Finish the routine by sitting comfortably, closing your eyes, and allowing your head to gently lower.
- Focus on your breath, inhaling and exhaling slowly.
- Release any remaining tension in your neck and shoulders, enjoying a few moments of relaxation.

Throughout these practices, remind seniors to move slowly, breathe mindfully, and modify any movement as needed for their individual comfort and ability. The key is to encourage gentle, controlled motions to enhance flexibility and release tension in the neck and shoulders.

Neck Stretches and Mobility

Neck stretches and mobility exercises play a crucial role in chair yoga for seniors, promoting flexibility, reducing stiffness, and alleviating discomfort. Here's a comprehensive guide to incorporating effective neck stretches and mobility exercises into a complete chair yoga routine:

1 Neck Tilts:

- Maintain a straight back while sitting comfortably in a chair.
- Bring your ear close to your shoulder while you gently cock your head to one side.
- As you feel the stretch down the side of your neck, hold for 15 to 30 seconds.
- Repeat on the other side.

2 Neck Turns:

- While seated, slowly turn your head to one side as far as comfortably possible.
- Hold for 15-30 seconds, feeling the stretch in your neck and upper back.
- Repeat on the other side.

3 Neck Flexion and Extension:

- Start by looking straight ahead.
- Feel the back of your neck stretch as you slowly bring your chin up to your chest.
- Hold for 15-30 seconds.
- Slowly lift your head back up and tilt it slightly backward, feeling a stretch in the front of your neck.
- Hold for 15-30 seconds.

4 Neck Circles:

- Gently rotate your neck in a circular motion, moving clockwise for 30 seconds.
- Then, switch to counterclockwise rotations for another 30 seconds.
- This exercise helps improve the range of motion and flexibility in the neck.

5 Shoulder Rolls with Neck Integration:

- Combine shoulder rolls with gentle neck movements.
- Roll your shoulders forward and backward while incorporating slow and controlled neck tilts and turns.

6 Ear to Shoulder Stretch:

- Sit with a straight back and gently bring one ear towards the corresponding shoulder.
- Hold for 15-30 seconds, feeling the stretch on the opposite side of your neck.
- Repeat on the other side.

7 Seated Cat-Cow Stretch:

- Sit on the edge of your chair with hands on your knees.
- Inhale as you arch your back, lift your chest, and tilt your head back slightly.
- Exhale as you round your back, drop your chin to your chest, and feel a stretch in your neck.

8 Chin Tucks:

- Sit with a straight back and gently tuck your chin towards your chest.

- Hold for a few seconds, feeling a stretch in the back of your neck.

Remember to perform these stretches and mobility exercises slowly and with controlled movements. Encourage deep, relaxed breathing throughout to enhance the overall benefits. Regular practice of these neck stretches will contribute to improved mobility, reduced tension, and increased comfort for seniors engaging in chair yoga.

Shoulder Rolls and Releases

Shoulder rolls and releases are integral components of chair yoga for seniors, promoting flexibility, mobility, and relaxation. These gentle exercises specifically target the shoulders, providing relief from tension and enhancing overall well-being.

Shoulder Rolls:

1 **Seated Position:**

- Sit comfortably in a chair with your feet flat on the ground and your spine straight.
- Inhale as you lift your shoulders towards your ears, creating tension.

- Exhale and roll your shoulders backward in a circular motion, releasing tension as you lower them.
- Repeat this movement for several breath cycles, encouraging a smooth and controlled roll.

2 Forward and Backward Rolls:

- Inhale, rolling your shoulders forward in a circular motion.
- Exhale as you bring your shoulders backward in a circular motion.
- Focus on the fluidity of the movement and synchronize it with your breath for a calming effect.

3 Alternate Direction:

- Change the direction of the shoulder rolls, ensuring a balanced release of tension in different muscle groups.
- Encourage participants to maintain awareness of their breath and move with intention.

Shoulder Releases:

1 Neck and Shoulder Stretch:

- Inhale and lift your right arm overhead.

- Exhale and gently lean to the left, creating a stretch along the right side of the neck and shoulder.
- Hold for a few breaths, feeling the release.
- Repeat on the other side.

2 Cross-Body Stretch:

- Inhale and extend your right arm across your chest.
- Exhale and use your left hand to gently pull the right arm closer to your body.
- Hold the stretch, feeling the release in the shoulder.
- Repeat on the other side.

3 Arm Circles:

- Lift both arms to shoulder height.
- Inhale as you circle your arms forward, and exhale as you circle them backward.
- This dynamic movement helps release tension in the shoulders and promotes circulation.

4 Eagle Arms:

- Take a breath and raise your arms to the sides.
- Exhale and cross your right arm over the left, bringing the palms together.

- Hold the position, feeling a stretch between the shoulder blades.
- Repeat with the left arm crossing over the right.

5 Tips for Chair Yoga for Seniors:

- Emphasize the importance of gentle, controlled movements to avoid strain.
- Urge participants to pay attention to their bodies and adjust exercises accordingly.
- Incorporate deep, mindful breathing to enhance relaxation and focus.

Integrating these shoulder rolls and releases into a complete chair yoga routine for seniors can contribute significantly to their physical and mental well-being, fostering a sense of ease and flexibility.

CHEST OPENER POSES

Chair yoga for seniors can greatly benefit from chest opener poses, promoting flexibility, mobility, and improved posture. Here are some comprehensive chest opener poses suitable for a complete chair yoga routine:

1 **Seated Mountain Pose:**

- With your feet flat on the floor, take a comfortable seat in a chair.
- Inhale, lengthen your spine, and reach your arms overhead with palms facing each other.
- Interlace your fingers and stretch upward, opening your chest. Hold and breathe deeply.

2 **Seated Cat-Cow Stretch:**

- Sit on the edge of the chair, place hands on knees.
- Inhale arching your back, lifting your chest (Cow Pose).
- Exhale rounding your spine, bringing chin to chest (Cat Pose).
- Repeat, syncing breath with movement.

3 **Seated Eagle Arms:**

- Cross your right arm under the left, and then bring palms together.
- Lift elbows to shoulder height, feeling a stretch across your upper back.
- After a few breaths of holding, switch sides.

4   Seated Cow Face Pose Variation:

- Bring your right arm behind your back, palm facing away.
- Reach your left hand over your shoulder, trying to clasp fingers.
- If you can't reach, use a strap or hold onto a towel. Repeat on the other side.

5   Seated Twist with Arm Extension:

- Sit tall, twist to the right, placing your left hand on the right knee.
- Inhale and extend the right arm up, opening the chest.
- Hold, then switch sides.

6   Seated Backbend:

- With your fingers pointed down, place your hands on your lower back.
- Inhale, lift your chest, and gently arch your spine backward.
- Keep the neck neutral and hold the stretch.

7   Seated Heart Opener:

- Sit at the edge of the chair, interlace fingers behind your back.
- Inhale, straighten arms, and lift chest, squeezing shoulder blades together.

8 Seated Shoulder Opener:

- Clasp hands behind your back, straighten arms, and lift them slightly.
- Feel the stretch across your chest and shoulders.

Remember to encourage slow, controlled movements, and emphasize the importance of deep, mindful breathing in each pose. Always respect individual abilities and adapt poses as needed for the participants. Regular practice of these chest opener poses can contribute to improved upper body flexibility and overall well-being in seniors.

Seated Backbends for Posture

Seated backbends are a beneficial component of chair yoga for seniors, promoting improved posture and flexibility. These gentle stretches can be easily incorporated into a seated routine, providing numerous advantages for overall well-being.

Purpose of Seated Backbends:

Seated backbends primarily focus on opening up the chest and shoulders while strengthening the spine. This helps counteract the effects of prolonged sitting, enhancing posture and reducing stiffness commonly experienced by seniors.

Preparation and Safety:

Start with proper posture – sit comfortably on a stable chair with feet flat on the floor. Ensure the spine is tall and shoulders are relaxed. Emphasize smooth and controlled movements, avoiding any abrupt or forceful actions to prevent strain.

Basic Seated Backbend:

Inhale deeply, lifting the chest toward the ceiling. Arch the back gently while keeping the neck in line with the spine. Hold for a few breaths, feeling a stretch across the chest and front of the shoulders. Exhale slowly as you return to an upright position.

Variations for Adaptability:

Recognize individual limitations and offer variations. For instance, individuals with lower back issues may benefit from a more subtle backbend, while those with greater flexibility can explore deeper stretches.

Use of Props:

Props such as a small cushion or folded blanket can provide support and comfort during seated backbends. Placing a prop at the lower back can enhance the stretch without compromising safety.

Breathing Awareness:

Encourage synchronized breathing with movement. Inhale during the backbend to expand the chest, and exhale while returning to an upright position. This rhythmic breathing enhances relaxation and mindfulness.

Incorporate Seated Backbends into a Routine:

Integrate seated backbends into a comprehensive chair yoga sequence for seniors. Combine with other seated poses, gentle twists, and stretches to create a well-rounded practice that addresses various aspects of flexibility and mobility.

Benefits for Posture:

Regular practice of seated backbends contributes to improved posture by strengthening the muscles supporting the spine. This, in turn, helps alleviate back pain and discomfort associated with poor posture.

Promote Mind-Body Connection:

Emphasize the connection between body and mind during seated backbends. Encourage participants to be present in the moment, fostering a sense of mindfulness and relaxation.

Consultation with Healthcare Professionals:
Stress the importance of consulting healthcare professionals before beginning any exercise program, especially for seniors with pre-existing health conditions. This ensures that the chair yoga routine, including seated backbends, is tailored to individual needs and restrictions.

Seated backbends in chair yoga for seniors are a valuable tool for promoting posture, flexibility, and overall well-being. When executed mindfully and with adaptability in mind, these gentle movements contribute to a more active and comfortable lifestyle.

Promoting Respiratory Function

Chair yoga for seniors can be an excellent way to promote respiratory function while providing a gentle and accessible form of exercise. Incorporating specific movements and breathing exercises into a complete chair yoga routine can enhance lung capacity, improve circulation, and contribute to overall respiratory health.

1 Deep Breathing Techniques:

- Start the chair yoga session with deep breathing exercises. Breathe deeply through your nose, pushing the diaphragm apart, and then gently release the breath through pursed lips. This encourages better oxygen exchange and engages the respiratory muscles.

2 Seated Cat-Cow Stretch:

- Incorporate gentle spinal movements like the seated cat-cow stretch. Inhale while arching the back and lifting the chest, then exhale while rounding the spine. This promotes flexibility in the spine and encourages deep breathing.

3 Diaphragmatic Breathing:

- Integrate diaphragmatic breathing exercises where seniors focus on breathing into the diaphragm rather than shallow chest breathing. This helps improve the efficiency of the respiratory system.

4 Seated Forward Bend:

- Include the seated forward bend to stretch the back and open up the chest. Encourage seniors to breathe deeply in this position to enhance lung expansion.

5 Arm Raises with Breath:

- Combine arm raises with synchronized breathing. Inhale while raising the arms, and exhale while lowering them. This not only promotes better oxygen intake but also enhances shoulder mobility.

6 Chair Pavanamuktasana (Wind-Relieving Pose):

- Guide seniors through a modified version of the wind-relieving pose while seated. This helps in releasing any trapped air in the digestive system and promotes abdominal breathing.

7 Chest Opener:

- Incorporate chest-opening poses, like clasping hands behind the back and gently lifting the arms. This helps in expanding the chest and improving lung capacity.

8 Alternate Nostril Breathing:

- Introduce alternate nostril breathing for balance. This technique involves blocking one nostril while inhaling and exhaling through the other, promoting a sense of calmness and balanced respiratory function.

9 Mindful Breathing Meditation:

- Conclude the chair yoga session with a brief mindful breathing meditation. This can involve focusing on the breath and bringing awareness to each inhalation and exhalation.

10 Encourage Regular Practice:

- Emphasize the importance of regular chair yoga practice for seniors to experience long-term benefits in respiratory function. Consistency is key in promoting overall well-being.

By integrating these elements into a complete chair yoga routine, seniors can enjoy a gentle yet effective means of promoting respiratory function, enhancing lung capacity, and maintaining overall respiratory health.

Chapter Three

ENHANCING UPPER BODY MOBILITY

Arm, Wrist, and Hand Exercises

For a complete chair yoga routine tailored to seniors focusing on the arm, wrist, and hand exercises, consider incorporating the following exercises:

1. **Wrist Circles:**

    - Extend arms in front while seated.
    - Rotate wrists clockwise and counterclockwise in circular motions.
    - Repeat for 10-15 repetitions in each direction.

2. **Finger Stretch:**

    - Extend arms forward, palms facing down.
    - Slowly spread fingers apart, then bring them back together.

- Repeat 10-15 times, focusing on gentle stretching.

3. Wrist Flexor and Extensor Stretch:

- Extend one arm forward, palm facing down, fingers pointing towards the floor.
- Gently press down on the fingers with the opposite hand, feeling the stretch in the wrist and forearm.
- Hold for 15-20 seconds and switch sides.

4. Thumb Touch:

- Touch the tip of each finger to the tip of the thumb, creating an "O" shape with each finger.
- Repeat this movement several times, enhancing dexterity and mobility.

5. Bicep Curls with Light Weights:

- Hold a light weight in each hand.
- Perform seated bicep curls, lifting and lowering the weights.
- Aim for 10-15 repetitions, gradually increasing as strength improves.

6. Seated Shoulder Rolls:

- Sit comfortably with a straight back.
- Roll shoulders forward and backward in a circular motion, promoting flexibility and reducing stiffness.

7. Seated Tricep Dips:

- Place hands on the armrests, fingers pointing forward.
- Lift and lower the body, engaging triceps.
- Perform 10-15 reps, adjusting intensity as needed.

8. Gentle Hand Clenches:

- Make a fist, then open your fingers wide.
- Repeat this movement to strengthen hand muscles.
- Perform 10-15 repetitions.

9. Wrist Flexor Stretch:

- Extend one arm forward, palm facing up.

- Gently press down on the fingers with the opposite hand, stretching the wrist and forearm.
- Hold for 15-20 seconds and switch sides.

10. Rotation with a Soft Ball:

- Hold a soft ball in both hands.
- Rotate the wrists clockwise and counterclockwise, squeezing the ball gently.
- Perform for 10-15 repetitions in each direction.

Remember to encourage seniors to perform these exercises at their own pace, emphasizing gentle and controlled movements. Always prioritize comfort and safety, adjusting the intensity based on individual abilities. Consultation with a healthcare professional before starting any exercise program is advisable, especially for seniors with pre-existing conditions.

Promoting Flexibility and Strength

Promoting flexibility and strength through chair yoga for seniors involves incorporating a well-rounded set of exercises tailored to the unique needs and limitations of older individuals. Here's a comprehensive overview:

1   Gentle Warm-Up:

- Begin with seated neck stretches, shoulder rolls, and wrist circles to warm up joints.
- Incorporate deep, mindful breathing to promote relaxation and focus.

2   Seated Side Stretches:

- Encourage lateral movement by gently reaching arms overhead and leaning to each side, promoting flexibility in the spine.

3   Chair Tadasana (Mountain Pose):

- Instruct seniors to sit tall, grounding their feet and reaching arms overhead, engaging core muscles for strength.

4   Seated Forward Fold:

- Promote hamstring flexibility and lower back release by guiding participants to hinge at the hips and reach towards their toes.

5 Chair Pigeon Pose:

- Improve hip flexibility and strength by guiding seniors to cross one ankle over the opposite knee while sitting, gently pressing on the crossed knee.

6 Seated Twist:

- Enhance spinal mobility with seated twists, encouraging seniors to rotate their torso while holding onto the back of the chair.

7 Leg Lifts:

- Strengthen leg muscles by lifting one leg at a time, holding briefly, and then lowering it down, repeating on both sides.

8 Chair Squats:

- Promote lower body strength by guiding seniors to stand up slightly from the chair and then sit back down, maintaining good posture.

9 Seated Balance Exercises:

- Incorporate leg lifts and ankle circles while seated to improve balance and stability.

10 Modified Sun Salutations:

* Adapt traditional yoga sequences to a
  seated position, including modified versions
  of sun salutations, promoting overall
  flexibility and strength.

11 Breathing and Meditation:

* Integrate mindful breathing exercises and
  short meditation sessions to enhance
  mental well-being and focus.

12 Cool Down:

* Finish the session with gentle stretches and
  relaxation techniques, such as seated chest
  openers and deep breathing exercises.

13 Safety Guidelines:

* Emphasize the importance of listening to
  their bodies, avoiding overexertion, and
  using the chair for support as needed.

14 Progression:

* Encourage seniors to gradually progress in
  intensity and duration as they become more
  comfortable with the exercises, ensuring a

safe and gradual improvement in flexibility and strength.

By combining these elements in a structured chair yoga routine, seniors can experience enhanced flexibility, improved strength, and overall well-being, all within the comfort and safety of a seated position.

Addressing Common Concerns

1. Limited Mobility:

- **Approach:** Chair yoga is specifically designed for seniors with limited mobility. It involves gentle movements and stretches that can be comfortably executed while seated, ensuring inclusivity for individuals with varying levels of mobility.
- **Benefits:** By focusing on seated poses, chair yoga promotes joint flexibility and muscle engagement without putting excessive strain on the body. This makes it an ideal choice for seniors who may struggle with traditional yoga poses due to restricted mobility.

2. Balance Issues:

- **Incorporating Support:** Seniors often face challenges with balance, increasing the risk of falls. Chair yoga incorporates poses that provide additional support, enabling participants to hold positions with greater stability.
- **Enhancing Safety:** The use of a chair as a prop during standing poses ensures that even those with balance issues can partake in the practice without compromising safety. This reduces the fear of falling and encourages participation.

3. Joint Pain and Stiffness:

- **Gentle Movements:** Chair yoga focuses on gentle movements that cater to seniors with joint pain and stiffness. These movements help increase joint mobility, promoting a gradual improvement in flexibility without causing discomfort.
- **Adaptability:** Instructors can adapt poses to accommodate individuals with arthritis or other joint-related concerns. This adaptability ensures that seniors can experience the benefits of yoga without exacerbating existing joint issues.

4. Chronic Conditions:

- **Tailored Practices:** Chair yoga can be tailored to suit individuals with chronic conditions such as arthritis, osteoporosis, or hypertension. Instructors can modify sequences to address specific health concerns while still providing a holistic yoga experience.
- **Emphasis on Well-being:** The practice not only supports physical health but also emphasizes mental and emotional well-being, contributing to an overall improvement in the management of chronic conditions.

5. Cognitive Concerns:

- **Clear Instructions:** To cater to seniors with cognitive concerns, chair yoga instructors use clear and simple instructions. This ensures that participants can follow along easily, promoting engagement and reducing potential confusion.
- **Repetitive Movements:** Some chair yoga routines incorporate repetitive movements, which can be beneficial for individuals with cognitive challenges by providing a structured and familiar practice.

6. Breathing Difficulties:

- **Breath-Centered Practices:** Chair yoga places a significant emphasis on controlled breathing exercises. This can benefit seniors with respiratory issues, helping improve lung capacity and respiratory function.
- **Adapted Breathing Techniques:** Instructors can modify breathing techniques to suit individual needs, making chair yoga accessible for those with varying degrees of respiratory challenges.

7. Fear of Falling:

- **Building Confidence:** Chair yoga provides a supportive environment that allows seniors to gradually build confidence in their movements. The chair serves as a stable prop, alleviating fears associated with balance-related incidents.
- **Gradual Progression:** Instructors often incorporate a gradual progression in difficulty, allowing participants to advance at their own pace and overcome the fear of falling over time.

8. Adaptability:

- **Individual Modifications:** Chair yoga is highly adaptable, allowing instructors to modify poses based on individual needs and limitations. This adaptability ensures that participants can engage in the practice comfortably and safely.
- **Variety of Poses:** The versatility of chair yoga allows for a wide variety of poses and movements, catering to individuals with different levels of fitness, flexibility, and health conditions.

9. Social Isolation:

- **Community Setting:** Chair yoga classes provide a social setting where seniors can connect with others who share similar health and wellness goals. This community aspect helps combat social isolation, promoting a sense of belonging and camaraderie.
- **Inclusive Environment:** The inclusive nature of chair yoga fosters a supportive community where participants can share their experiences and support one another, contributing to overall well-being.

10. Limited Space:

- **Convenience:** Chair yoga can be performed in confined spaces, making it suitable for seniors living in small homes or assisted living facilities. The minimal equipment required adds to the convenience of practicing chair yoga in various settings.
- **Accessibility:** The accessibility of chair yoga, both in terms of space and equipment, ensures that seniors can easily incorporate it into their daily routines, regardless of living arrangements.

Chair yoga addresses a spectrum of common concerns for seniors, ranging from physical limitations to social and environmental factors. Its adaptability, safety features, and holistic approach make it an inclusive and beneficial practice for enhancing the overall well-being of the senior population.

IMPROVING POSTURE

Improving posture through chair yoga for seniors involves a holistic approach that focuses on flexibility, strength, and mindful awareness. Here's a comprehensive guide:

1. Seated Mountain Pose:

- Sit tall in a chair with feet flat on the floor.
- Engage core muscles and extend the spine upward.
- Relax shoulders and elongate the neck.
- Breathe deeply, promoting awareness of the body's alignment.

2. Seated Forward Bend:

- Hinge at the hips, reaching hands towards the floor.
- Keep the spine straight and lengthened.
- Feel a gentle stretch in the back and hamstrings.
- Maintain steady breath to enhance the stretch.

3. Seated Twist:

- Sit with feet planted, twist the upper body to one side.
- Hold onto the back of the chair for support.
- Rotate the torso, stretching the spine.
- Repeat on the other side for balance.

4. Chest Opener:

- Interlace fingers behind the back, straighten arms.
- Lift the chest, opening the shoulders.
- Expand the chest while keeping the spine aligned.

- Encourage seniors to breathe deeply for increased oxygen flow.

5. Seated Cat-Cow Stretch:
- Sit tall, inhale arching the back (Cow Pose).
- Exhale, round the back (Cat Pose).
- Move through the poses with breath, enhancing spinal flexibility.
- Promotes a healthy range of motion in the spine.

6. Neck Stretches:
- Gently tilt the head to one side, holding for a few breaths.
- Repeat on the other side.
- Perform forward and backward neck stretches.
- Encourage slow and controlled movements to prevent strain.

7. Seated Warrior Pose:
- Bend the other knee and extend one leg forward.
- Align the spine and lift arms overhead.
- Engage core muscles for stability.
- Switch legs to balance the stretch on both sides.

8. Mindful Breathing:
- Emphasize the importance of deep, diaphragmatic breathing.

- Inhale through the nose, expanding the abdomen.
- Exhale slowly through pursed lips, promoting relaxation.
- Connect breath with movement to enhance mind-body awareness.

9. Seated Meditation:
- End the session with a few minutes of seated meditation.
- Focus on posture, breathing, and cultivating a sense of calm.
- Encourage seniors to maintain an upright, comfortable position.

10. Regular Practice:
- Stress the importance of consistent practice.
- Gradually progress intensity to build strength and flexibility.
- Remind seniors to listen to their bodies and modify poses as needed.

By incorporating these chair yoga exercises into their routine, seniors can enhance posture, flexibility, and overall well-being in a safe and accessible manner.

Chapter Four

STRENGTHENING CORE AND LOWER BODY

Seated Twists and Abdominal Engagement

Instructions

1. **Starting Position:** Sit comfortably on a stable chair, feet flat on the ground, and hands resting on your thighs.
2. **Spinal Alignment:** Inhale deeply, lengthening the spine, and ensuring a tall, upright posture.
3. **Twisting Motion:** Exhale slowly as you initiate the twist, gently rotating your upper body to one side.
4. **Hand Placement:** Place one hand on the opposite knee and the other on the backrest or armrest for support.
5. **Breathing:** Hold the twist for a few breaths, inhaling to lengthen the spine and exhaling to deepen the twist.

6. **Return to Center:** Inhale as you return to the center, then repeat the twist on the other side.

Benefits:

- **Spinal Flexibility:** Seated twists enhance the flexibility of the spine, reducing stiffness and promoting a greater range of motion.
- **Digestive Support:** The twisting motion stimulates abdominal organs, aiding digestion and potentially relieving discomfort.
- **Stress Relief:** Gentle twists release tension in the back and shoulders, contributing to overall stress reduction.

Modifications:

For those with limited mobility, consider holding onto the sides of the chair and focusing on the rotation of the upper body within a comfortable range.

Abdominal Engagement in Chair Yoga

Instructions:

1. **Seated Posture:** Sit with an upright posture, shoulders relaxed, and hands resting on your thighs.

2. **Inhale and Engage:** Inhale deeply, then engage the abdominal muscles by gently drawing the navel toward the spine.
3. **Breath Control:** Hold the engagement for a few seconds, maintaining a controlled breath without holding it excessively.
4. **Exhale and Release:** Exhale slowly, allowing the abdominal muscles to relax.
5. **Repeat Gradually:** Gradually increase the duration of abdominal engagement over subsequent practices.

Benefits:

- **Core Strength:** Abdominal engagement builds strength in the core, offering stability and support for daily activities.
- **Posture Improvement:** Strengthening the abdominal muscles contributes to improved posture, reducing the risk of back discomfort.
- **Mindful Breathing:** The practice encourages breath awareness, fostering mindfulness and relaxation.

Modifications:

Seniors can customize the intensity of abdominal engagement based on their comfort level, ensuring a controlled and safe practice.

Safety Tips:

1. **Listen to Your Body:** Perform these exercises at a pace that feels comfortable, avoiding any movements causing discomfort or pain.
2. **Proper Alignment:** Emphasize gentle, controlled movements during seated twists to maintain proper spinal alignment and prevent strain.
3. **Consultation:** Before starting a new exercise routine, especially for seniors with pre-existing conditions, consult with a healthcare professional.

Incorporating seated twists and abdominal engagement into chair yoga for seniors provides a comprehensive approach to physical well-being. Regular practice not only enhances flexibility and core strength but also contributes to a sense of relaxation and vitality in the senior population.

Core-Strengthening Sequences

Chair yoga for seniors can incorporate effective core-strengthening sequences to promote stability and enhance overall well-being. Here's a comprehensive guide to core-strengthening chair yoga:

1. Seated Cat-Cow Stretch:

- Sit upright with feet flat on the floor.
- Inhale, arching the back and lifting the chest (Cow).
- Exhale, rounding the spine, tucking the chin to the chest (Cat).
- Repeat slowly, engaging core muscles for stability.

2. Seated Knee Lifts:

- Sit tall and lift one knee towards the chest.
- Hold briefly, engaging the core.
- Lower the foot and switch to the other knee.
- Repeat in a controlled manner.

3. Twisting Chair Pose:

- Sit with feet flat, hands on opposite knees.
- Inhale, lengthen the spine.
- Exhale, twist to one side, placing the opposite hand on the back of the chair.
- Hold for a few breaths, engaging the core.
- Repeat on the other side.

4. Seated Leg Raises:

- Sit at the edge of the chair.
- Lift one leg straight, engaging the core.
- Hold briefly before lowering.
- Alternate legs, maintaining control.

5. Seated Side Stretch:

- Inhale, reaching arms overhead.
- Exhale, leaning to one side, engaging the obliques.
- Inhale back to center and repeat on the other side.

6. Chair Plank:
- Hold onto the sides of the chair, walk feet back.
- Keep your head and heels in a straight line..
- Engage the core and hold for 20-30 seconds.

7. Seated Boat Pose:
- Sit at the edge of the chair, lean back slightly.
- Lift legs, creating a V shape.
- Hold, engaging abdominal muscles.
- Lower feet with control.

8. Seated Mountain Pose:
- Sit tall, reaching arms overhead.
- Engage the core, lifting the ribcage.
- Hold, focusing on breath and stability.

9. Seated Bicycle Crunches:
- Sit comfortably, hands behind the head.
- Lift one knee towards the chest, twisting to bring the opposite elbow towards it.
- Alternate sides in a controlled, bicycle-like motion.

10. Chair Warrior Pose:
- Extend one leg back, keeping it straight.
- Bend the front knee, engaging the core for stability.
- After a few breaths of holding, switch sides.

These chair yoga sequences aim to enhance core strength, stability, and flexibility for seniors. Always encourage slow, controlled movements and remind participants to listen to their bodies. It's advisable to consult with a healthcare professional before starting any new exercise routine, especially for seniors or individuals with pre-existing health conditions

Engaging Abdominal Muscles

Engaging abdominal muscles in chair yoga for seniors is fundamental for fostering core strength, stability, and overall well-being. This comprehensive approach involves a series of seated poses and mindful movements tailored to the needs of older individuals.

1 Seated Posture and Breath Awareness:

- Start with a comfortable seated position, feet flat on the floor, and spine erect.

- Inhale deeply, expanding the chest, and exhale while gently drawing the navel toward the spine.
- Encourage seniors to maintain a steady and controlled breath throughout the practice.

2 Mindful Breathing and Movement Integration:

- Emphasize synchronizing breath with movement to enhance awareness.
- For example, during inhalation, seniors can lengthen their spine, and during exhalation, engage the abdominal muscles.

3 Seated Twists:

- Incorporate gentle seated twists to promote spinal flexibility and activate the core.
- Instruct participants to initiate the twist from the abdomen, gradually moving the torso without straining.

4 Seated Forward Bends:

- Explore seated forward bends with an emphasis on abdominal engagement.
- Participants can hinge at the hips, reaching towards their toes while maintaining a strong core connection.

5 **Leg Lifts and Knee-to-Chest Exercises:**

- Integrate exercises targeting the lower abdominals, such as seated leg lifts or bringing knees toward the chest.
- Stress the importance of controlled movements to prevent strain on the lower back.

6 **Pelvic Tilts:**

- Incorporate pelvic tilts, where participants gently rock back and forth on their sitting bones.
- This movement engages and releases the abdominal muscles, promoting improved posture and alleviating lower back discomfort.

7 **Seated Boat Pose Variations:**

- Gradually introduce variations like seated boat pose, encouraging seniors to lift one or both legs while maintaining a strong core.
- Provide support with props like cushions if needed, ensuring accessibility for all participants.

8 Mind-Body Connection:

- Encourage seniors to focus on the sensations in their abdominal region, fostering a deeper mind-body connection.
- Remind them to listen to their bodies and modify poses as necessary.

9 Use of Props for Added Resistance:

- Integrate props such as resistance bands or small weights to add gentle resistance, enhancing the effectiveness of abdominal engagement exercises.

10 Relaxation and Closing Poses:

- Conclude the session with relaxation poses, such as seated meditation or deep breathing exercises.
- This allows seniors to experience the holistic benefits of chair yoga, promoting a sense of calmness and heightened body awareness.

Regular practice of this comprehensive chair yoga routine not only strengthens the abdominal muscles but also contributes to improved balance, reduced back pain, and increased overall mobility for seniors. It creates a supportive and inclusive environment, emphasizing the importance of adapting the practice to individual abilities and needs.

Pelvic Tilts

Pelvic tilts are a beneficial exercise in chair yoga for seniors, promoting flexibility and stability in the pelvic region. To perform pelvic tilts while seated, start by sitting upright in a sturdy chair with feet flat on the floor. Place your hands on your knees.

1. **Inhale and Engage:** Take a deep breath in and engage your abdominal muscles. This creates a stable foundation for the movement.

2. **Tilt Forward (Anterior Pelvic Tilt):** As you exhale, gently tilt your pelvis forward, arching your lower back. The front of your hips should feel stretched. This movement helps improve posture and flexibility in the lower spine.

3. **Tilt Backward (Posterior Pelvic Tilt):** Inhale again and slowly tilt your pelvis backward, rounding your lower back. This motion stretches the muscles in the lower back and enhances mobility.

4. **Repeat the Sequence:** Continue alternating between anterior and posterior pelvic tilts for several breaths. The controlled, rhythmic movement helps improve circulation, reduce stiffness, and enhance the range of motion in the pelvic area.

5. **Modify as Needed:** Seniors with mobility or balance concerns can perform seated pelvic tilts, ensuring a safe and effective practice. The support of the chair provides stability while still offering the benefits of the exercise.

6. **Awareness of Sensations:** Encourage seniors to pay attention to the sensations in their lower back and hips during the pelvic tilts. If any discomfort arises, they should adjust the intensity or consult with a healthcare professional.

7. **Integration into Routine:** Incorporate pelvic tilts into a comprehensive chair yoga routine for seniors. Combine with other seated exercises, breathing techniques, and gentle stretches to create a well-rounded practice that addresses various aspects of physical well-being.

8. **Consistency is Key:** Regular practice of pelvic tilts contributes to improved pelvic

flexibility, core strength, and overall spinal
health. Encourage seniors to include this
exercise consistently in their chair yoga
routine for optimal benefits.

By integrating pelvic tilts into chair yoga for seniors,
you provide a gentle yet effective way for them to
enhance flexibility, maintain pelvic health, and
promote overall well-being in a safe and accessible
manner.

LOWER BODY FLEXIBILITY

Lower body flexibility is a crucial aspect of chair
yoga for seniors, promoting overall mobility, joint
health, and a sense of well-being. Designing a
comprehensive routine involves incorporating a
variety of seated and standing poses that target
different muscle groups in the lower body.

1 Seated Warm-Up:

- Begin with gentle warm-up exercises to
  prepare the lower body. Include ankle
  circles, knee lifts, and hip rotations to
  increase blood flow and loosen the joints.
- Encourage participants to maintain a tall
  spine and engage in controlled, deep
  breathing throughout the warm-up to
  promote relaxation.

2 Seated Forward Bends:

- Seated forward bends are effective for stretching the hamstrings, lower back, and improving overall flexibility. Guide seniors to reach forward toward their toes while keeping the back straight.
- Use cushions or props to support those with limited flexibility, ensuring a comfortable and safe experience.

3 Seated Hip Openers:

- Incorporate seated hip-opening poses such as the seated pigeon pose. This helps to release tension in the hips and improve flexibility.
- Emphasize the importance of moving within one's range of motion, avoiding any discomfort or strain.

4 Standing Chair Poses:

- Transition to standing chair poses to further engage the lower body muscles. Chair squats are excellent for building strength and flexibility in the thighs and glutes.
- Guide participants to use the chair for support, ensuring stability and confidence in their movements.

5 Leg Stretches:

- Integrate seated and standing leg stretches
  to target the quadriceps and calf muscles.
  Seated leg lifts and standing leg extensions
  are beneficial for enhancing flexibility in
  these areas.
- Emphasize the extension of the legs while
  keeping the movements controlled and
  mindful.

6 Breathing and Relaxation:

- Throughout the session, emphasize the
  importance of proper breathing. Deep,
  mindful breaths can enhance relaxation and
  contribute to improved flexibility.
- Conclude the routine with a brief relaxation
  period, allowing participants to focus on
  their breath and experience the benefits of
  the practice.

7 Modifications and Individualization:

- Encourage seniors to listen to their bodies
  and make modifications based on their
  individual needs and comfort levels.
- Provide variations for each pose, ensuring
  that participants can tailor the practice to
  their unique abilities and constraints.

By incorporating these elements into a chair yoga routine, seniors can experience a comprehensive and accessible approach to enhancing lower body flexibility, contributing to improved physical and mental well-being. Regular practice can lead to increased range of motion, reduced stiffness, and an overall sense of vitality.

Seated Leg Stretches

Seated leg stretches are crucial components of chair yoga for seniors, promoting flexibility, circulation, and overall well-being. These gentle exercises can be performed while sitting comfortably, making them accessible for individuals with limited mobility.

1 Seated Forward Bend:

- With your feet flat on the ground, take a lofty seat in a firm chair.
- Inhale, lengthen your spine, and as you exhale, hinge at your hips, reaching towards your toes.
- Hold the stretch, feeling a gentle pull in your hamstrings and lower back.
- Repeat several times, maintaining a slow and controlled pace.

2 Knee to Chest Stretch:

- Sit with feet flat, lift one knee towards your chest, holding behind the thigh.
- Gently pull the knee closer to your chest, feeling a stretch in the hip and lower back.
- Hold briefly, then switch legs.
- This stretch helps improve hip flexibility and releases tension in the lower back.

3 Seated Leg Lifts:

- Sit upright, extend one leg straight in front of you, keeping the foot flexed.
- Lift the leg a few inches off the floor and hold briefly.
- Lower the leg back down without letting it touch the floor.
- This exercise strengthens the quadriceps and improves circulation in the legs.

4 Ankle Circles:

- Raise one foot off the floor and move your ankle in a circle.
- Perform both clockwise and counterclockwise movements.
- Switch to the other foot.
- Ankle circles enhance ankle flexibility and alleviate stiffness.

5   Inner Thigh Stretch:

- Open your legs wider than hip-width apart while seated.
- Gently press on the inner thighs with your hands, feeling a stretch in the groin area.
- Hold the stretch, then release.
- This exercise targets the inner thigh muscles and improves hip flexibility.

6   Seated Calf Stretch:

- Extend one leg straight with the heel on the floor.
- Flex the foot towards you, feeling a stretch in the calf.
- After a few breaths of holding, switch legs.
- This stretch helps prevent calf tightness and enhances ankle mobility.

7   Seated Pigeon Pose:

- Cross one ankle over the opposite knee, maintaining a straight back.
- Gently press on the crossed knee, feeling a stretch in the outer hip.
- Hold the pose and switch sides.
- The seated pigeon pose releases tension in the hips and improves hip joint flexibility.

Encourage seniors to perform these seated leg stretches regularly, emphasizing the importance of deep breathing and mindfulness during each movement. Always prioritize comfort and encourage modifications based on individual needs and abilities.

Ankle and Foot Exercises

Chair yoga for seniors is a great way to promote flexibility, strength, and overall well-being. When focusing on ankle and foot exercises within this context, it's essential to prioritize safety and comfort. Here's a set of ankle and foot exercises suitable for chair yoga:

1 **Toe Taps:**

- Sit comfortably in the chair with feet flat on the floor.
- Lift and tap your toes on the ground, engaging your ankle muscles.
- Repeat for 10-15 taps, gradually increasing as strength improves.

2 **Ankle Circles:**

- Raise one foot off the floor and turn your ankle in a clockwise and counterclockwise direction.
- Perform 8-10 circles in each direction, then switch to the other foot.

3 Heel Raises:

- Keep your feet flat on the floor and lift your heels off the ground.
- After holding for a short while, release the pressure.
- Repeat 10-15 times to strengthen calf muscles.

4 Toe Point and Flex:

- Extend one leg and point your toes, then flex them back towards you.
- After ten repetitions, move to the other foot.

5 Alphabet with Your Feet:

- Imagine drawing the alphabet with your toes while keeping your heel on the ground.
- This helps in improving ankle mobility and flexibility.

6 Resistance Band Exercises:

- Secure a resistance band around the ball of your foot and gently flex and point your foot against the resistance.
- Perform 10-15 repetitions on each foot.

7 Foot Massage:

- Roll a small ball (tennis ball, for example) under your foot to massage the arch and relieve tension.

8 Seated Leg Lifts:

- While sitting, lift one leg straight out in front of you, engaging your quadriceps and ankle muscles.
- Hold for a few seconds and lower the leg.
- Repeat 10-15 times on each leg.

9 Ankle Dorsiflexion Stretch:

- With one foot flat on the ground, take a seat on the chair's edge.
- Gently press the toes towards your shin until you feel a stretch in the front of your ankle.
- After 15 to 30 seconds of holding, move to the other foot.

10 Calf Stretch:

- While seated, extend one leg straight out and flex the foot, feeling a stretch in the calf.
- After 15 to 30 seconds of holding, move to the opposite leg.

Remember to encourage seniors to move within their comfort zone, modify exercises as needed, and always consult with a healthcare professional before starting any new exercise routine. Regular practice of these ankle and foot exercises can contribute to improved stability and mobility.

Gentle Knee Movements

Gentle knee movements play a crucial role in a complete chair yoga routine tailored for seniors. These exercises focus on enhancing flexibility, improving joint mobility, and promoting overall well-being. Here's a comprehensive guide:

1 Seated Knee Lifts:

- Begin by sitting comfortably in a chair with feet flat on the floor.
- Lift one knee towards your chest, holding for a few seconds.
- Lower the leg gradually, then switch to the other side.
- This movement improves circulation and flexibility in the knee joint.

2 Knee Extensions:

- Sit with your back straight and extend one leg forward, keeping it straight.
- After a brief moment of holding, lower the leg.
- Repeat with the other leg.
- This exercise helps strengthen the quadriceps and improves knee stability.

3 Chair Knee Circles:

- Place your feet flat on the ground when you sit.
- Lift one knee and make circular motions with your foot, clockwise and then counterclockwise.
- This movement promotes synovial fluid circulation in the knee joint, reducing stiffness.

4 Seated Leg Swings:

- While seated, swing one leg forward and backward, keeping it straight.
- Repeat on the other leg.
- This dynamic movement enhances flexibility in the knee and hip joints.

5 Ankle-to-Knee Stretch:

- Form a figure-four by crossing one ankle over the other knee.
- Gently press down on the raised knee to feel a stretch in the outer hip and knee.
- Switch to the other side.
- This stretch improves flexibility in the hips and relieves tension in the knee area.

6 Seated Heel Slides:

- Sit with your back straight and slide one heel along the floor towards your body.
- Hold briefly, then extend the leg.
- Repeat with the other leg.
- This movement helps maintain flexibility in the knee joint and stretches the hamstrings.

7 Seated Knee Flexor Stretch:

- Sit at the edge of the chair and extend one leg forward.
- Gently pull your toes towards you, feeling a stretch in the back of the knee.
- Switch to the other leg.
- This stretch targets the muscles behind the knee, enhancing flexibility.

8 Chair Squats:

- Place your feet shoulder-width apart in front of the chair.
- Lower your body as if sitting back into the chair, keeping knees aligned with your toes.
- Stand back up.
- This exercise strengthens the muscles around the knee joint and promotes stability.

9 Seated Knee Hugs:

- While seated, hug one knee towards your chest.
- Hold for a moment, then switch to the other leg.
- This movement gently stretches the lower back and increases knee flexibility.

Incorporating these gentle knee movements into a chair yoga routine for seniors can contribute significantly to joint health, mobility, and overall comfort. Always encourage participants to move within their comfortable range of motion and consult with a healthcare professional before starting any new exercise program.

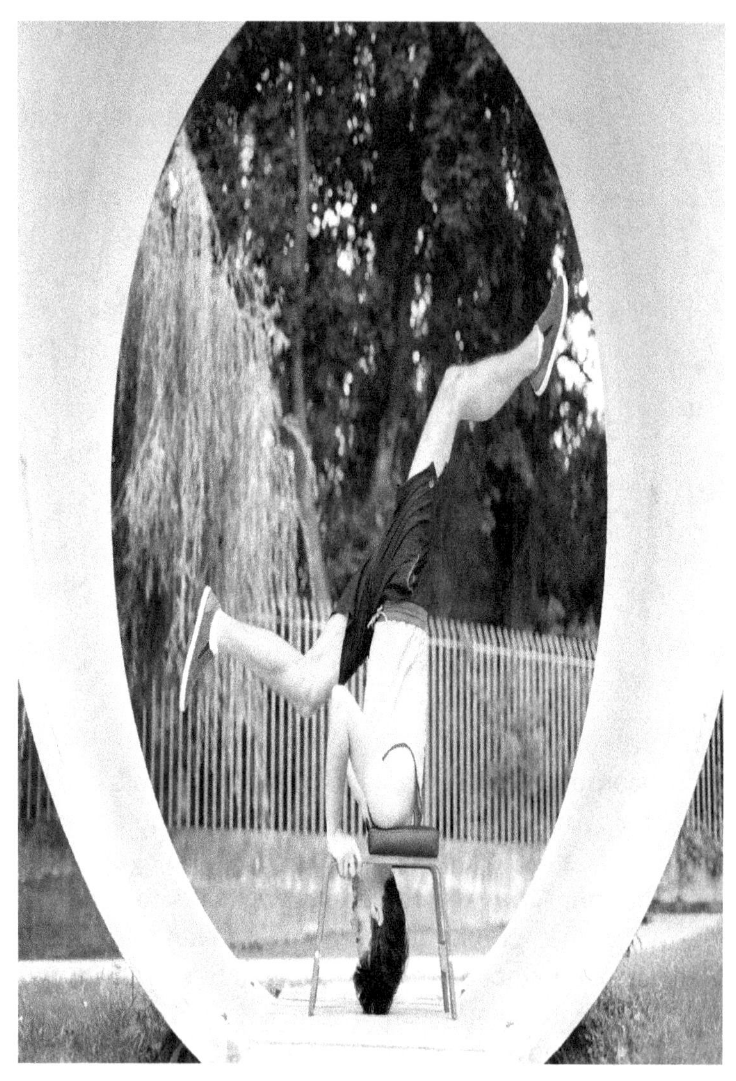

Chapter Five

BALANCE, STABILITY, AND RELAXATION

Chair Yoga for Balance

Chair yoga for seniors focuses on promoting balance, flexibility, and overall well-being while accommodating individuals who may have mobility limitations. This gentle form of yoga is practiced sitting on a chair or using it for support, making it accessible for seniors or those with physical challenges.

1. Seated Mountain Pose:

- Comfortably sit with your feet flat on the ground.
- Arms raised aloft, palms facing each other, inhale.
- Engage core muscles and stretch upward.
- Hold for a few breaths, promoting good posture.

2. Seated Forward Bend:

- Hinge at the hips and lean forward, reaching towards the floor.
- Keep the back straight and feel the stretch in the hamstrings.
- Hold for a comfortable duration while breathing deeply.

3. Seated Side Stretch:

- Inhale, lift arms overhead, and clasp hands.
- Lean gently to one side, elongating the spine.
- Feel the stretch along the side of the torso.
- Repeat on the other side.

4. Chair Cat-Cow Stretch:

- Sit on the edge of the chair with hands on knees.
- Inhale, arch the back (Cow), lifting the chest.
- Exhale, round the spine (Cat), dropping the chin.
- Repeat the sequence to enhance spinal flexibility.

5. Seated Warrior Pose:

- Extend one leg straight, foot flexed.

- Bend the opposite knee, placing the foot flat on the floor.
- Raise arms overhead, stretching upward.
- Switch legs and repeat for balance.

6. Seated Leg Lifts:

- Sit upright and extend one leg straight.
- Raises the leg to a few inches above the ground.
- Hold briefly, engaging the muscles.
- Lower and switch to the other leg.

7. Chair Twist:

- Sit with your spine straight, cross one leg over the other.
- Inhale and lengthen the spine.
- Exhale, twisting towards the crossed leg.
- Repeat on the other side to enhance spine mobility.

8. Ankle Rolls and Toe Taps:

- Lift feet off the floor and rotate the ankles in both directions.
- Tap toes on the floor for a gentle foot exercise.
- Enhances ankle mobility and helps prevent stiffness.

9. Diaphragmatic Breathing:

- Sit comfortably and focus on deep, diaphragmatic breathing.
- Inhale through the nose, expanding the belly.
- Exhale through pursed lips, engaging the core.
- Promotes relaxation and reduces stress.

10. Guided Meditation:

- Finish with a brief meditation, focusing on mindfulness.
- Encourages mental relaxation and a sense of calm.

A senior's healthcare professional should be consulted before beginning any exercise program. Chair yoga for balance not only improves physical health but also fosters a sense of peace and mindfulness, contributing to a holistic well-being for seniors.

Balancing Poses with Support

Chair yoga for seniors can incorporate a variety of balancing poses with support to enhance stability and flexibility. These poses are designed to be gentle, considering the limitations that seniors may have. Here's a comprehensive guide to balancing poses with support in chair yoga for seniors:

1. **Seated Mountain Pose:**
    - Sit tall in the chair, feet flat on the ground.
    - Engage core muscles and reach arms overhead, palms facing each other.
    - This promotes spinal alignment and improves posture.

2. **Seated Side Stretch:**
    - Inhale, raising arms overhead.
    - Exhale, gently leaning to one side, stretching the side body.
    - Repeat on the other side.

3. **Seated Knee Lifts:**
    - With your back straight, sit at the chair's edge.
    - Lift one knee towards the chest and hold briefly.
    - Lower and switch legs.
    - Improves balance and strengthens leg muscles.

4. **Seated Leg Extension:**
    - Extend one leg forward, keeping it elevated.

- Hold for a few breaths, engaging thigh muscles.
- Switch legs, promoting strength and flexibility.

5. **Seated Tree Pose:**
   - Place the outer edge of one foot on the inner thigh of the opposite leg.
   - Hold onto the back of the chair for support.
   - Enhances balance and opens the hip.

6. **Seated Warrior Pose:**
   - Extend one leg back with toes pointing down.
   - Keep the opposite knee bent at a 90-degree angle.
   - Use the chair for balance.
   - Strengthens legs and improves stability.

7. **Seated Eagle Arms:**
   - Cross one arm over the other, bringing palms together.
   - Lift elbows and reach arms away.
   - This seated version promotes shoulder flexibility and balance.

8. **Seated Cat-Cow Stretch:**
    - Inhale arching the back, lifting the chest.
    - Exhale rounding the spine.
    - Promotes flexibility in the spine and gentle core engagement.

9. **Seated Forward Bend:**
    - Hinge at the hips and reach forward with a straight back.
    - Hold onto the chair legs for support.
    - Stretches the hamstrings and promotes relaxation.

10. **Seated Twist:**
    - Sit tall and twist the upper body to one side, holding onto the back of the chair.
    - Repeat on the other side.
    - Aids in spinal mobility and digestion.

Always encourage seniors to listen to their bodies, move slowly, and modify poses as needed. These chair yoga balancing poses with support provide a safe and effective way for seniors to enhance physical well-being while enjoying the benefits of yoga.

Tips for Safe Balance Practices

1. Consultation with Healthcare Professionals:
Before seniors embark on a chair yoga routine, it's crucial for them to consult with healthcare professionals to ensure that the exercises align with their health conditions and limitations.

2. Appropriate Chair Selection:
Choose a stable, non-slip chair without wheels. The ideal chair allows seniors to place their feet flat on the ground, ensuring a solid foundation for balance poses.

3. Comprehensive Warm-Up:
Begin the session with a thorough warm-up. Gentle movements increase blood circulation, warm the muscles, and prepare the body for the ensuing chair yoga routine, reducing the risk of strains or injuries.

4. Mindful Breathing Practices:
Emphasize the importance of mindful breathing throughout the session. Deep and intentional breathing not only enhances relaxation but also serves as a focal point during balance poses.

5. Focus on Core Strengthening:
Integrate exercises that target core strength. A strong core is fundamental for stability, and incorporating seated twists and abdominal

contractions helps enhance this crucial aspect of balance.

6. Proper Use of Support:

Encourage the use of the chair as a support mechanism during standing poses or balance exercises. Gradually, participants can reduce dependency on the chair as their balance improves.

7. Avoiding Overexertion:

Remind participants to listen to their bodies and not push themselves beyond their comfort levels. Overexertion can lead to fatigue and compromise the safety of the practice.

8. Individualized Pose Adaptations:

Chair yoga should be adaptable to individual abilities. Provide modifications for poses to accommodate different levels of flexibility, strength, and mobility among participants.

9. Integration of Props:

Utilize props such as yoga blocks or cushions to offer additional support or modify poses. Props can make the practice more accessible and comfortable for seniors with varying physical abilities.

10. Controlled and Gradual Movements:

Advocate for slow and controlled movements to enhance stability. Rapid or sudden movements may disrupt balance and increase the risk of falls.

11. Mindful Transitions between Poses:

Highlight the importance of mindful transitions between poses. Encourage participants to move deliberately, avoiding abrupt changes that may compromise their balance.

12. Eye Focus Techniques:

Teach participants to fix their gaze on a stationary point during balancing poses. This helps improve concentration, focus, and overall stability during the practice.

13. Incorporation of Seated and Standing Balances:

Create a well-rounded practice that includes a mix of seated and standing balance poses. Seated poses offer stability, while standing poses challenge balance and improve overall strength.

14. Consistency in Practice:

Stress the significance of regular and consistent chair yoga practice. Over time, this can lead to improvements in strength, flexibility, and balance, ultimately reducing the risk of falls.

15. Thoughtful Cool-Down:

Conclude the session with gentle stretches and a thoughtful cool-down. This aids in relaxing the muscles, promoting flexibility, and ensuring a smooth transition back to a resting state.

Remember, these tips should be viewed as general guidelines, and individual considerations must be taken into account. Always prioritize safety, encourage participants to move within their comfort zones, and celebrate progress at each individual's pace.

RELAXATION AND DEEP BREATHING

Relaxation and deep breathing are crucial components of chair yoga for seniors, offering numerous benefits such as stress reduction, improved mood, and increased self-awareness. The following exercises are designed to help seniors practice relaxation and deep breathing while seated in a chair:

1. **Breathwork and Meditation:** Focus on a simple yet effective breathwork and meditation exercise for seniors, as demonstrated in this YouTube video. This exercise involves taking slow, deep breaths, inhaling through the nose and exhaling through the mouth.

2. **Seated Posture:** Sit comfortably in your chair with your feet flat on the floor and your

hands on your thighs. Extend your back, raise your chest slightly, and roll your shoulders back. Shut your eyes or look forward gently.

3. **Coherent Breathing:** While seated, push down into the chair with your lower body and buttocks, while lifting your chest and neck and head up tall, feeling like you are stretching the spine. Pretend there is a big balloon attached to the crown of your head, pulling your head and upper body straight up. Your head is level, your eyes looking across the room. Try to focus on some point across the room. Spend a few minutes holding this stance while paying attention to your breathing while sitting.

4. **Overhead Stretch:** While still seated in the chair, take a deep breath through your nose and raise both arms above your head, hands together over your head. As you exhale, slowly lower your arms, the palms of your hands together, in front of your heart. Repeat this a few times slowly inhaling while you raise both arms and exhaling as you lower them

These exercises can be easily completed at home or in a group, combining breathing awareness with gentle yoga exercises that can be done while sitting in a chair. Wearing loose clothing and having a yoga mat or non-slip rug to stand on can enhance the practice. It is essential to consult with a healthcare provider before starting chair yoga to receive guidance on poses that are best for you and your health

Deep Breathing Techniques

Deep breathing techniques can be combined with chair yoga poses for seniors to create a relaxing and mindful practice. Here are some exercises that can be easily done at home or in a group setting:

1. **Coherent Breathing:** This technique aims to be aware of your breath and breathe slowly while mentally counting the lengths of your inhales and exhales. Begin by counting to 2 as you inhale, pause, and exhale to the count of 2. As you become more comfortable, you can work up to longer breaths, counting to 3, 4, 5, or 6 as you inhale or exhale

2. **Breathing and Chair Yoga:** Focus on yoga breathing to aid in stress reduction, enhance mental clarity, and improve overall emotional well-being. Inhale deeply and feel your body relax into a seated position with your hands on your belly, noticing the sensations of breathing

3. **Seated Yoga Flow, Breathing & Chair Yoga for Seniors:** This class offers a seated yoga and chair yoga routine designed specifically for elderly seniors and older adults. It aims to maintain a healthy and active lifestyle, reduce stress, and promote a sense of inner peace

4. **Chair Yoga for Seniors & Mindful Breathing:** This video provides a gentle and mindful chair yoga practice, focusing on breathwork and meditation exercises for seniors

5. **Chair Yoga | Beginners Breathwork & Meditation for Seniors:** This video offers a simple yet effective breathwork and meditation exercise for seniors, focusing on a seated position with hands on the belly

6. **Yoga Breath & Meditation Sequence - Chair Yoga for Seniors:** This sequence from Stronger Seniors® Chair Yoga Program combines deep breathing with yoga poses for seniors, promoting relaxation and a sense of well-being

When practicing these techniques, it is essential to wear loose clothing, preferably untucked, and any type of clothing is fine. Just don't do that exercise if you are in any pain. All yoga exercises should be gentle, never pushing the body, and the goal is to feel relaxed and peaceful

Guided Relaxation and Meditation

Guided relaxation and meditation play a crucial role in complete chair yoga for seniors, providing physical and mental benefits.

1. Stress Reduction:
Guided relaxation techniques help seniors release tension and reduce stress. Incorporating deep breathing exercises and mindfulness meditation during chair yoga sessions can promote a sense of calmness and relaxation.

2. Improved Mental Health:
Regular meditation has been linked to improved mental well-being. For seniors, this is particularly beneficial in reducing symptoms of anxiety and depression, enhancing overall mood, and fostering a positive outlook on life.

3. Enhanced Mobility:

Meditation combined with chair yoga can improve flexibility and mobility. Guided relaxation allows seniors to focus on gentle movements, promoting joint flexibility and muscle strength, which are vital for maintaining mobility as they age.

4. Mind-Body Connection:

Guided relaxation fosters a stronger mind-body connection. Seniors can learn to be more aware of their bodies, promoting better balance, coordination, and a heightened sense of body awareness, which is crucial for preventing falls and injuries.

5. Pain Management:

Meditation techniques incorporated into chair yoga can aid in pain management. Seniors dealing with chronic pain conditions may find relief through mindfulness practices, helping them cope with discomfort and improve their overall quality of life.

6. Sleep Improvement:

Seniors often face challenges with sleep. Guided relaxation before bedtime can assist in calming the mind, reducing insomnia, and promoting better sleep quality. This is vital for overall health and daytime functionality.

7. Social Interaction:

Chair yoga sessions that include guided relaxation provide a social setting for seniors. The communal aspect of participating in meditation with peers fosters a sense of community and connection, addressing feelings of isolation and loneliness.

8. Cognitive Benefits:

Meditation has been associated with cognitive benefits, including improved focus and memory. For seniors, engaging in guided relaxation exercises can contribute to maintaining cognitive function and potentially slowing down cognitive decline.

9. Adaptability for Physical Limitations:

Chair yoga, incorporating guided relaxation and meditation, is adaptable for seniors with physical limitations. The seated postures make it accessible for those who may have difficulty with traditional yoga poses, allowing everyone to enjoy the benefits of these practices.

10. Holistic Well-being:

Incorporating guided relaxation and meditation into chair yoga for seniors promotes a holistic approach to well-being. It addresses physical, mental, and emotional aspects, contributing to a comprehensive wellness strategy for the aging population.

Chapter Six

ADAPTING AND IMPLEMENTING CHAIR YOGA

Modifying Poses for Different Abilities

Modifying poses in chair yoga for seniors is crucial to accommodate varying abilities and ensure a safe and enjoyable practice. Here's a comprehensive guide on modifying poses for different abilities:

1 **Seated Mountain Pose:**

- For those with limited mobility, encourage a gentle modification by having them sit comfortably with their feet flat on the floor.
- Use cushions or folded blankets to provide extra support for individuals with lower back issues.

2   **Chair Forward Bend:**

- Suggest a gentle forward lean for participants with flexibility concerns, ensuring they focus on a comfortable stretch rather than reaching too far.
- Offer the option of resting forearms on thighs for added support.

3   **Seated Twist:**

- Emphasize gentle twists to accommodate seniors with back issues, allowing them to go only as far as feels comfortable.
- Provide variations like holding onto the chair for stability during the twist.

4   **Chair Warrior Poses:**

- Simplify Warrior poses by incorporating a seated leg lift or stretch instead of standing variations.
- Encourage participants to engage core muscles for stability during these modified seated Warrior poses.

5   **Chair Tree Pose:**

- Modify Tree Pose by having seniors place the sole of their foot on the inner calf or

ankle, rather than the thigh, for better
balance and stability.

- Suggest using the back of the chair for
additional support if needed.

6 Seated Cat-Cow Stretch:

- Guide participants to perform a seated
version of Cat-Cow, focusing on gentle
spinal flexion and extension while seated
comfortably.
- Emphasize breath awareness to enhance
the benefits of the stretch.

7 Chair Sun Salutation:

- Break down Sun Salutation into seated
components, such as seated mountain
pose, forward bend, and gentle twists,
allowing seniors to experience the flow in a
seated position.
- Encourage smooth transitions between
poses to maintain a fluid practice.

8 Seated Meditation:

- Make meditation accessible by suggesting
comfortable seated positions with proper
support.

- Utilize props like cushions or blankets to enhance comfort during meditation sessions.

9 Breathing Exercises:

- Integrate breathing exercises into the practice, emphasizing the importance of deep, controlled breaths for relaxation.
- Offer options for those with respiratory concerns, such as pursed lip breathing or diaphragmatic breathing.

10 Individualized Guidance:

- Always provide individual attention and modifications based on each participant's unique abilities and needs.
- Encourage open communication, allowing seniors to express any discomfort or concerns during the practice.

By tailoring chair yoga poses to different abilities, seniors can experience the physical and mental benefits of yoga in a safe and inclusive manner. Regularly assess participants' comfort levels and adjust modifications accordingly to promote an enjoyable and accessible chair yoga practice.

Tailoring Practices for Individuals

Tailoring chair yoga for seniors involves adapting traditional yoga practices to suit the unique needs and limitations of older individuals. Here's a comprehensive guide on tailoring chair yoga for seniors:

1 Assessment and Individualization:

- Begin by assessing each senior's physical abilities, flexibility, and any existing health concerns.
- Tailor the chair yoga routine based on individual needs, modifying poses accordingly.

2 Chair Selection:

- Choose stable and supportive chairs without arms for better movement.
- Ensure chairs are positioned on a non-slip surface to prevent accidents.

3 Warm-up and Joint Mobility:

- Incorporate gentle warm-up exercises to prepare the body for movement.

- Focus on joint mobility exercises to improve flexibility and reduce stiffness.

4 Breathing Techniques:

- Emphasize deep breathing exercises to enhance lung capacity and promote relaxation.
- Teach seniors to synchronize breath with movement to improve mind-body connection.

5 Seated Poses:

- Modify classic yoga poses to be performed while seated on the chair.
- Include poses that work on balance, strength, and flexibility, such as seated twists, forward bends, and side stretches.

6 Adaptive Modifications:

- Offer variations and modifications for each pose to accommodate different ability levels.
- Use props like blocks or cushions to support seniors in maintaining proper alignment.

7 Mindfulness and Relaxation:

- Integrate mindfulness and meditation practices to reduce stress and enhance mental well-being.
- Encourage guided relaxation techniques to promote a sense of calm.

8 Safety Precautions:

- Emphasize the importance of listening to their bodies and not pushing beyond their limits.
- Instruct seniors to use the chair for support when needed to prevent falls or strain.

9 Incorporate Therapeutic Elements:

- Include elements of therapeutic yoga, such as gentle massage or self-myofascial release using a tennis ball, to alleviate tension.

10 Catering to Health Conditions:

- Consider common health conditions like arthritis or osteoporosis and tailor poses accordingly.
- Consult with healthcare professionals to ensure the yoga routine aligns with any medical recommendations.

11 Encourage Consistency:

- Stress the benefits of consistent practice in improving overall physical and mental well-being.
- Provide resources and encouragement for seniors to continue their practice outside of class.

12 Feedback and Adjustment:

- Regularly collect feedback from participants to make necessary adjustments to the chair yoga routine.
- Be adaptable and responsive to individual needs and progress.

By incorporating these tailored practices, chair yoga for seniors can become a safe, enjoyable, and effective way to enhance their physical and mental health.

Working with Props and Tools

When creating a complete chair yoga routine for seniors, it's essential to carefully select props and tools that enhance safety, accessibility, and comfort. Here's a comprehensive guide:

Props:

1. **Chair:**
   - Choose a sturdy, armless chair with a flat seat and a backrest.
   - Ensure the chair is placed on a non-slip surface for stability.

2. **Yoga Straps:**
   - Assist seniors in achieving stretches by providing additional length.
   - Useful for modifications, making poses more accessible.

3. **Yoga Blocks:**
   - Support alignment and balance for various poses.
   - Place under hands or feet to reduce strain and enhance stability.

4. **Blankets:**
   - Offer padding and comfort during seated or lying poses.
   - Can be folded or rolled to provide additional support.

5. **Bolsters:**
   - Enhance relaxation and comfort during seated or reclined poses.
   - Support the spine and promote proper alignment.

6. **Resistance Bands:**
   - Aid in gentle strength training.
   - Improve flexibility and provide resistance for arm exercises.

7. **Eye Pillow:**
   - Foster relaxation during meditation or Savasana.
   - Helps seniors unwind and release tension.

Tools:

1. **Instructional Materials:**
   - Provide clear, written or verbal instructions for each pose.
   - Include diagrams or images for visual guidance.

2. **Music and Ambient Sounds:**
   - Create a calming atmosphere during the practice.
   - Choose soft music or nature sounds to enhance the experience.

3. **Timer or Stopwatch:**
   - Set specific durations for poses to avoid overexertion.
   - Helps seniors pace themselves and enjoy a gradual practice.

4. **Personalized Modifications:**
   - Be prepared to offer variations for individuals with different abilities.
   - Ensure that each participant feels comfortable and supported.

5. **Communication Tools:**
   - Establish a clear line of communication with participants.
   - Use a microphone if necessary, and encourage feedback.

6. **Safety Precautions:**
   - Have a first aid kit on hand.
   - Ensure the space is well-lit and free of obstacles.

7. **Documentation:**
   - Maintain records of participants' health concerns and limitations.
   - Keep emergency contact information readily available.

Remember, the key to a successful chair yoga session for seniors lies in adaptability. Regularly assess the participants' needs and adjust the props and tools accordingly, promoting a safe and enjoyable experience for everyone.

CHAIR YOGA ROUTINES

Chair yoga is a gentle form of yoga adapted to be performed while sitting on a chair or using a chair for support. It's particularly beneficial for seniors, providing a safe and accessible way to improve flexibility, strength, and overall well-being. Here's a comprehensive guide to chair yoga routines for seniors:

1 Seated Mountain Pose:

- Pose with your back straight and your feet flat on the ground.
- Breathe in and raise your arms, palms facing each other.
- Exhale, bringing hands down to the heart center.
- Repeat for a few breaths, promoting mindfulness and alignment.

2 Neck Stretches:

- Gently tilt your head to one side, holding for a few breaths.
- Repeat on the other side.
- Slowly move your head forward and backward, promoting neck flexibility.

3 Seated Forward Bend:

- Sit forward on the chair, feet flat.
- Inhale, lengthen the spine; exhale, hinge at the hips, reaching towards your toes.
- Hold for a few breaths, feeling a stretch in the hamstrings and lower back.

4 Chair Cat-Cow Stretch:

- Sit with hands on knees.
- Inhale, arch the back (Cow); exhale, round the spine (Cat).
- Repeat, promoting spinal flexibility and relieving tension.

5 Seated Twist:

- Sit with feet flat, twist to one side, placing one hand on the opposite knee and the other on the chair back.
- After a few breaths of holding, switch sides.
- This helps improve spine mobility and aids digestion.

6 Leg Extensions:

- Sit forward on the chair, extend one leg straight, flexing the foot.
- After holding for a few breaths, swap your legs.

- Promotes leg strength and flexibility.

7 Chair Warrior Pose:

- Sit with feet hip-width apart.
- Inhale, raise arms overhead, bringing palms together.
- Exhale, bend elbows, bringing hands to the back.
- This helps in strengthening the arms and shoulders.

8 Ankle Rolls:

- Lift one foot, rotate the ankle clockwise and then counterclockwise.
- Repeat with the other foot.
- Enhances ankle flexibility and improves circulation.

9 Deep Breathing Exercises:

- Sit comfortably, inhale deeply through the nose, exhale through the mouth.
- Focus on breath awareness, promoting relaxation and reducing stress.

10 Meditation and Mindfulness:

- Finish the routine with a few minutes of seated meditation.

- Encourage seniors to focus on their breath or practice guided meditation for relaxation.

Always ensure that seniors listen to their bodies, modify poses as needed, and consult with a healthcare professional before starting any new exercise routine. Regular chair yoga practice can contribute to improved balance, flexibility, and a sense of well-being for seniors.

Morning Energizer, Midday Relaxation, and Evening Wind-Down

The Complete Chair Yoga for Seniors is a program designed to provide a gentle and relaxing yoga practice that can be done in the morning, midday, and evening. These sessions aim to promote energy, relaxation, and stress relief for seniors. Here are the details for each session:

Morning Energizer
The morning session is designed to invigorate and energize participants for the day ahead. It may include:

- Gentle stretches and strengthening exercises to improve flexibility and balance

- Breathing exercises to promote relaxation and focus
- Mindfulness meditation to set intentions for the day

Midday Relaxation

The midday session is tailored to help participants unwind and relax during the day. It may include:

- Seated meditation with guided imagery to promote calming and stress relief
- Gentle yoga postures to stretch and release tension
- Breathing exercises to help balance and focus

Evening Wind-Down

The evening session is designed to help participants unwind and prepare for sleep. It may include:

- Guided meditation to reduce anxiety and stress
- Restorative yoga postures to stretch and relax the body
- Breathing techniques to enhance calmness and enhance the quality of sleep
- Optional use of singing bowls or other calming sounds

By incorporating these chair yoga sessions into your daily routine, seniors can enjoy the benefits of yoga at any time of the day. The program is adaptable and can be modified to suit individual needs and preferences.

Customizing Routines for Personal Needs

Customizing routines for personal needs in chair yoga for seniors involves creating a practice that is gentle, supportive, and tailored to individual abilities. Here are some suggestions for designing a chair yoga routine for seniors:

1. **Warm-up:** Begin with a few minutes of gentle breathing exercises and stretches to warm up the body and prepare for the practice. This can include seated breathing, neck rolls, and shoulder stretches.

2. **Seated Postures:** Choose seated postures that are comfortable and accessible for seniors. Some examples include seated forward bending, seated twist, and seated lunge. Modify these postures as needed to accommodate different levels of mobility and flexibility.

3. **Stretches:** Incorporate a mix of stretches targeting different muscle groups, such as hamstrings, quadriceps, and hip flexors. These can be done in various ways, such as seated, standing, or lying down. Ensure that the stretches are gentle and not overly intense to avoid injury.

4. **Strength Exercises:** Include seated exercises to strengthen key muscle groups, such as the core, back, and shoulders. These can be done using body weight or light resistance, such as a resistance band or small weights.

5. **Balance and Coordination:** Incorporate exercises to improve balance and coordination, such as seated single-leg stands or seated crane poses. These exercises can help improve proprioception and coordination.

6. **Relaxation:** End the practice with a few minutes of relaxation, such as seated meditation or deep breathing exercises. This will help seniors to calm the mind and release tension from the body.

When designing a chair yoga routine for seniors, it is essential to consider the individual's abilities and needs. Encourage participants to listen to their bodies and modify poses as necessary to ensure a comfortable and effective practice. Additionally, it is crucial to provide clear instructions and demonstrations for each exercise to ensure proper form and technique.

Overcoming Challenges

Overcoming challenges in chair yoga for seniors involves addressing mobility, balance, and stability issues. Here are some tips and strategies to help seniors overcome these challenges and enjoy the benefits of chair yoga:

1. **Choose the right chair:** Use a stable, comfortable, and sturdy chair with a backrest and armrests for support. Ensure that the chair is at the right height, allowing for comfortable seated positions and easy movement.

2. **Seek professional guidance:** For seniors new to chair yoga, it's essential to consult a physical therapist or yoga instructor to ensure proper form and avoid overexertion. They can provide guidance on modifying poses and exercises to suit individual needs and abilities.

3. **Practice proper form:** Maintain good posture and form throughout the practice to avoid strain or injury. Focus on smooth, controlled movements and breathe deeply and slowly during each pose

4. **Use props:** Utilize props such as blankets, cushions, or straps to help with balance, stability, and flexibility. These can be placed under the feet, knees, or shoulders to provide additional support and comfort.

5. **Modify poses:** Adapt poses to suit individual needs and abilities by using different variations or modifications. For example, seniors with limited mobility can use a chair for support during standing poses or opt for seated variations of poses that require standing

6. **Focus on balance and stability:** Incorporate exercises that challenge balance and stability, such as seated forward bends, pigeon poses, and eagle arms. These exercises can help improve posture and prevent falls.

7. **Monitor your progress:** Keep track of your progress and adjust exercises as needed. Be patient and consistent in your practice,

and remember that it's essential to listen to your body and avoid overexertion

8. **Address individual needs:** Be mindful of any pre-existing health conditions or limitations and adjust your practice accordingly. Consult with a healthcare professional to determine which exercises are safe and appropriate for your specific needs.

By following these tips and strategies, seniors can overcome challenges in chair yoga and enjoy the numerous benefits of this accessible form of exercise. Regular practice can lead to improved strength, flexibility, balance, and mental well-being

Embracing the Benefits and Regular Practice

Embracing the benefits and regular practice of chair yoga for seniors can lead to a healthier and more active lifestyle. Chair yoga is a gentle form of exercise that focuses on stretching, breathing, and meditation, making it suitable for individuals with mobility limitations or those who want to improve their overall well-being. Some of the key benefits and advantages of chair yoga for seniors include:

1. **Improved flexibility:** Chair yoga helps to stretch the body in areas that may not be normally stretched, increasing flexibility and maintaining overall mobility for daily tasks

2. **Strengthened muscles:** Through various poses, chair yoga can help build and strengthen muscles, which can improve balance, coordination, and mobility, as well as protect the body from injury

3. **Enhanced balance and coordination:** Chair yoga can help improve balance and coordination, reducing the risk of falls and promoting overall stability

4. **Reduced joint pain:** Regular practice of chair yoga can help alleviate joint pain, making it an ideal form of exercise for individuals with arthritis or other joint conditions

5. **Reduced fear of falling:** Chair yoga can help seniors build confidence and reduce the fear of falling, as it provides a supportive environment for practicing yoga poses

6. **Stress reduction:** The combination of stretching, deep breathing, and meditation in chair yoga can help alleviate stress, lower

blood pressure, and improve mental well-being

7. **Increased circulation and energy levels:** Regular practice of chair yoga can improve circulation, leading to increased energy levels and a sense of well-being

To get started with chair yoga, seniors can participate in group classes, follow online videos, or practice with the help of a physical therapist or yoga instructor. It is essential to consult with a healthcare professional before starting any new exercise program, especially for individuals with pre-existing health conditions or concerns. By incorporating chair yoga into their daily routine, seniors can enjoy numerous health benefits and lead a more active and fulfilling lifestyle.

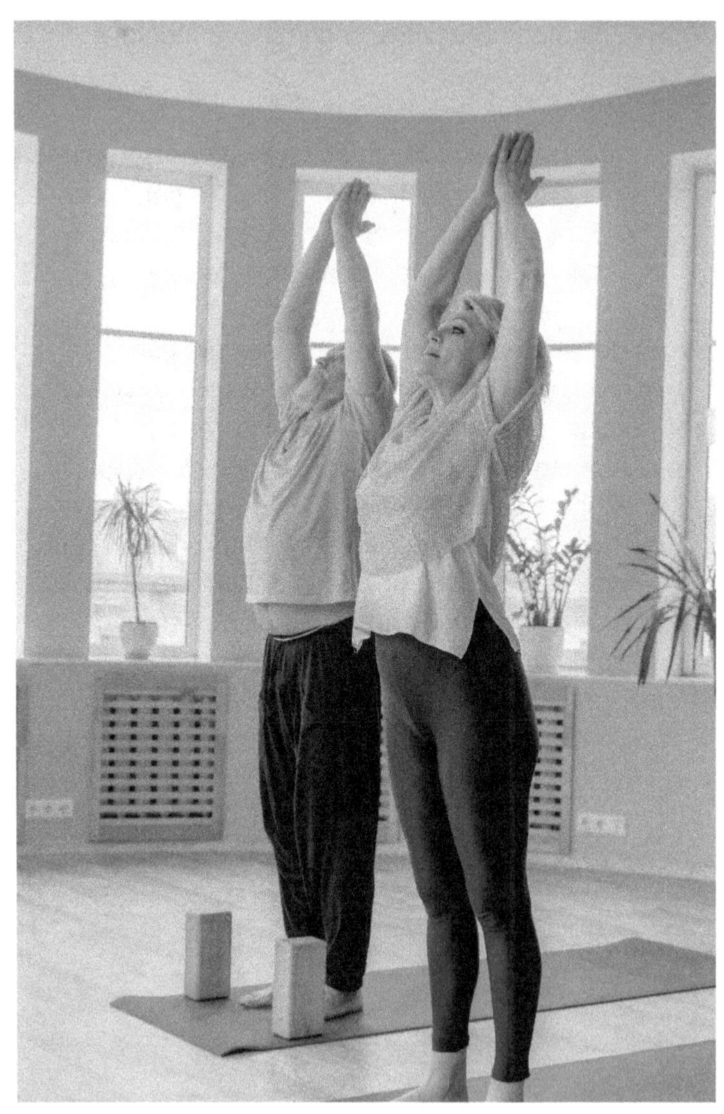

CONCLUSION

Our exploration of Chair Yoga for seniors, it is evident that this holistic approach to wellness extends far beyond the confines of a physical exercise routine. The amalgamation of gentle movements, intentional breathing, and mindful awareness encapsulates a comprehensive strategy for promoting not just physical health, but also mental and emotional well-being.

Throughout our journey, we've delved into a myriad of seated poses designed to enhance flexibility, improve posture, and increase overall strength. Yet, beyond the tangible benefits lies a profound connection between body and mind. The slow, deliberate motions, coupled with conscious breathing, create a symbiotic relationship that fosters a sense of tranquility and inner peace.

As seniors engage in Chair Yoga, they are not merely performing physical exercises; they are partaking in a therapeutic ritual that nurtures the body, calms the mind, and uplifts the spirit. The emphasis on adaptability and accessibility ensures that individuals of varying fitness levels and physical abilities can partake in this enriching practice, making it truly inclusive.

Moreover, the impact of Chair Yoga extends beyond the immediate physical benefits. It becomes a tool for self-discovery and self-care, empowering seniors to embrace their bodies, acknowledge their strengths, and navigate the aging process with grace and resilience. The cultivation of mindfulness throughout the practice encourages participants to live in the present moment, appreciating the beauty of the now.

In this concluding reflection, let us celebrate the essence of Chair Yoga as more than just a series of exercises but as a transformative journey toward holistic well-being. May the seniors who embark on this path find not only improved physical health but also a profound sense of balance, vitality, and enduring serenity. As we bid farewell to our exploration of Chair Yoga for seniors, let it stand as a testament to the timeless wisdom that wellness is a harmonious dance between the body, mind, and soul.